HOT TOPICS IN SPORTS AND ATHLETICS

HOT TOPICS IN SPORTS AND ATHLETICS

SAMUEL R. BAKERE
EDITOR

Nova Science Publishers, Inc.
New York

Library of Congress Cataloging-in-Publication Data

Hot topics in sports and athletics / Samuel R. Bakere, editor.
p. cm.
ISBN 978-1-60456-077-0 (hardcover)
1. Sports. 2. Athletics. I. Bakere, Samuel R.
GV565.H68 2007
796--dc22

2007045948

Published by Nova Science Publishers, Inc. ✢ New York

Contents

Preface

Sports and athletics are at once big business, spectator sports, body conditioning, mind expanding and it has been said form the only pages of most newspapers which are truthful and without political agendas. This new book presents articles which are of current interest in the field.

Chapter 1 - These studies examined the effects of sport-related advertising on body image. In Study 1, two hundred and twenty four collegiate females were categorised into regular exercisers and non-exercisers. In the pre-test and post-test (i.e., before and after exposure to advertising), each participant completed the Silhouette Measure of Body Image (SMBI; Stunkard, Sorenson and Schlusinger, 1983), the 9-item Social Physique Anxiety Scale (Martin, Rejeski, Leary, McAuley and Bane, 1997) and the Attitudes Towards Sport Advertisements (ATSA; adapted by Sabiston and Monroe, 2001, from Rabak-Wagner, Eickoff-Shemek and Kely-Vance, 1998), and the exercisers completed the 7-subscale Reasons for Exercise Inventory (Silberstein, Striegel-Moore, Timko and Rodin, 1988). They were then assigned to the model or product-related advertising condition. Participants were shown 15 sport-related advertisements either showing models (model condition) or workout shoes (product condition). Participants were given five minutes to view the advertisements, and then completed the questionnaires again. The results showed that the exercisers who were exposed to the model condition scored significantly ($p<.01$) higher on all measures in the post-test compared to the pre-test. The non-exercisers exposed to the model condition increased significantly ($p<.05$) on all measures from pre- to post-test but scored significantly ($p<.05$) lower on all post-test measures than the exerciser group. The product condition groups did not increase significantly on any measure ($p>.05$ in all cases). In Study 2, two hundred and forty nine sedentary undergraduates (126 males, 123 females) completed the SPAS, the SMBI and the ATSA. Following the pre-test, participants were shown 15 sport-related same-sex advertisements. Participants were given five minutes to view the advertisements, before completing the measures again. Group x test ANOVAs revealed that, in both the pre-test and the post-test, females scored significantly ($p<.05$) higher than males on the SMBI and SPAS. The SMBI, SPAS and ATSA scores of the female participants, and the SPAS and ATSA scores of the males, increased significantly ($p<.05$) from pre- to post-test. Males' SMBI scores were higher in the post-test than the pre-test but the difference was not statistically significant ($p>.05$). These results show that the use of very fit and toned models in the advertising of sport-related products can have a detrimental effect upon body image of both males and females.

Chapter 2 - Athletes are at increased risk for eating disorders (ED). Eating disorders in athletes may have severe physical and mental consequences, including failure to attain peak bone mass, low-trauma fractures and stress fractures, vertebral instability and curvature, prolonged psychological difficulties with weight and food, and even death. The high prevalence and unique nature of ED in athletes have led researchers to describe athlete-specific syndromes, including anorexia athletica and the female athlete triad of disordered eating, menstrual irregularity, and osteopenia/osteoporosis. Eating disorders in athletes have distinct etiologies and require specialized approaches to diagnosis, prevention, and treatment. Research on ED in athletes has increased dramatically in the past two decades, following the rapid increase in women's participation in athletics; however, many gaps remain in the authors understanding. Participation in weight-dependent sports may also account for a considerable proportion of ED in men, but male athletes have not been well studied. This chapter will critically review the latest research on ED in athletes, including: (1) issues in the measurement of ED, including the female athlete triad; (2) sport-and gender-specific prevalences; (3) risk and protective factors; (4) short and long-term sequelae; (5) prevention strategies; and (6) treatment strategies, including a review of pharmacologic agents to prevent or treat osteopenia and osteoporosis. This chapter will identify gaps in the current research and recommend directions for future research.

Chapter 3 - The chapter intends to examine the consumer attitude towards ATHENS 2004 Olympic Products, their purchasing behavior, as well as, the impact of the various means of promotion on their attitude and purchasing behavior. ATHENS 2004 Olympic Products are more than simple souvenir products. They bear the ATHENS 2004 emblem and its characteristics, representing the visual identity of the ATHENS 2004 Olympic Games The research results lead to certain useful conclusions on Sports Marketing, which may be used either by existing sports organizations with their organized marketing departments or on future large-scale sports events, such as the Beijing 2008 Olympic Games.

Chapter 4 - The current study addressed two research questions. First, study 1 examined whether spectators' mood before they were exposed to a losing game (i.e., pre-game mood) influenced their mood after the game (post-game mood) and their information processing. Secondly, study 2 examined whether the influence of pre-game mood found in Study 1 was modified by personal relevance (i.e., team identification) with a sporting game. The results indicated that pre-game mood influenced participants' post-game mood and information processing system. The results of the second study also supported the hypotheses that post-game mood and spectators' information processing were influenced by pre-game mood and personal relevance (i.e., team identification). As hypothesized, two-way interaction between pre-game mood and personal relevance was found in post-game mood whereas no interaction was found in information processing. This study was able to identify a group of people who were more affected by the result of home game and who were more effectively responded to mood manipulation.

Chapter 5 - Problems of usage of steroids and other performance enhancing drugs in professional and amateur athletics have been the focus of a series of investigative hearings before the House Government Reform Committee. The Committee began taking evidence on

March 17, 2005, when several former and current players, medical experts, and major league baseball executives were summoned to testify in the first hearing. Committee Chairman Tom Davis has urged all sports leagues to "acknowledge that their testing programs need improvement" and has framed bipartisan legislation to establish a uniform testing policy for major professional sports leagues. Currently, there are four professional athletic drug testing bills before Congress: S. 1114 (Senator McCain); H.R. 2565 (Representative Davis); H.R. 1862 (Representative Stearns); and H.R. 2516 (Representative Sweeney). The McCain and Davis bills are virtually identical, and all four bills would establish minimum drug standards – including random testing – for some professional sports leagues.

Congressionally mandated drug-testing requirements for both public employees and workers in private industry subject to federal regulation have a fairly long and well established legal history. Nonetheless, the federal courts have recognized limits, largely anchored in constitutional privacy interests of affected workers, that circumscribe governmental authority to impose suspicionless random testing requirements in the public or private sectors. These decisions establish that "compelling" governmental interests may, in appropriate circumstances, override constitutional objections to testing procedures by employees whose privacy expectations are diminished by the nature of their duties or workplace scrutiny to which they are otherwise subject. They further suggest, however, that substantial constitutional difficulties probably confront any broad-based testing program that is not limited to specific occupational categories or to persons for whom the government is able to demonstrate some special need to test.

It could be argued that professional players have a diminished expectation of privacy as the consequence of league or association rules that already require routine physical examinations and testing for drugs in certain circumstances. Moreover, a separate argument could be made that safety and health concerns associated with steroid usage, and the importance of professional athletes as role models for the nation's youth, justify unannounced testing for anabolic steroids or other controlled substances. Testing of randomly selected athletes may also be the least intrusive route to an effective steroid detection program. Past major league baseball procedures, it has been argued, do not deter steroid use. Moreover, arguably, the reasonable suspicion standard may be unworkable since most often there may be no outward symptoms to signal the use of steroids.

Chapter 6 - The use of performance-enhancing substances by athletes has a long history, predating the ancient Greek Olympiads. Concern about this practice was manifested in the 20th century by, in the case of the Olympics, the creation of anti-doping organizations, and the adoption of anti-doping policies by these organizations and professional sports leagues in the United States. Leading the way was the International Olympic Committee (IOC), which implemented testing in 1968 at the Olympic Games in Grenoble, France, and Mexico City, Mexico. The National Basketball Association (NBA) and the National Football League (NFL) followed suit in the 1980s. Major League Baseball implemented an anti-drug policy in 2003.

This report compares current anti-doping policies for performance enhancing substances among the Olympic movement and three professional sports — Major League Baseball, the NBA, and the NFL. Details associated with each of the selected group's policy are presented in Table 1. The report also presents elements of what have been identified as model anti-doping policies and (in the appendix) provides a comparison of Major League Baseball's former and current anti-doping policies (Table 2) and a glossary of related terms.

In general, the report indicates that the anti-doping policies for the Olympic movement are more independent of the sports they regulate than are the policies of Major League Baseball, the NBA, and the NFL, both in the manner in which they are established and in the entities responsible for their implementation. For example, the World Anti-Doping Agency (WADA) unilaterally established the anti-doping policy for Olympic athletes, whereas the professional sports leagues' policies are the result of negotiations with their respective players associations. The Olympic movement also maintains the most comprehensive list of prohibited substances and methods, and provides sanctions that are more strict than in the professional sports. For example, the Olympic standard provides a two-year ban for a first violation, whereas Major League Baseball imposes a 10-day suspension without pay for a first violation. Also, Olympic athletes and NFL players are responsible for what is in their bodies, but neither Major League Baseball nor the NBA addresses this subject.

Direct comparison of these sports is sometimes difficult because the policies use different terminology or make reference to other standards. The policies are also constantly changing in response to the development of new substances that are sometimes designed to avoid detection. In some cases, the policies prohibit certain substances for which tests are not available in order to inform athletes about harmful substances. However, in other cases, tests and sanctions are not provided for substances for which tests are available. For example, except for "reasonable cause" testing, Major League Baseball's policy provides for testing and sanctions only with regard to steroids — not other substances prohibited in the league's policy.

This report will be updated as anti-doping policies change and elements of those policies become clearer.

Chapter 7 - The present study investigated the factorial validity of the Brunel Mood Scale for use with UK, Italian and Hungarian athletes. One thousand five hundred and eleven mood responses from athletes were analysed using Confirmatory Factor Analysis (CFA). CFA on the Italian, Hungarian and UK athletes were close to the .90 criterion for acceptable fit initially highlighted by Bentler (1990), but below the .95 fit index suggested by Hu and Bentler (1995). It is argued that CFA results lend some support for the proposed validity of an eight-factor and 32-item mood scale. However, as the fit index was marginal, further work was needed. Eight separate CFAs on each subscale indicated acceptable fit indices for each factor. As confusion is a cognitive rather than affective construct, the authors decided to remove confusion and re-analyse data on a 21-item and seven-factor scale. CFA results on the 21-item and seven-factor scale indicated fit indices over .90, hence an improvement over the 32-item version. In conclusion, the 21-item and 32-item BRUMS represent a theoretically and empirically supported approach to investigating mood for use in UK, Hungarian and Italian athletes.

Chapter 8 - In a neutral and controlled environment, physical performance during a short-duration exercise fluctuates during the day with an acrophase close to 18:00 h. The diurnal increase in muscle power is mainly attributed to a diurnal increase in muscle force. This diurnal increase in muscle force is mainly attributed to a diurnal increase in muscle contractile properties. Today, the physiological basis of this variation in muscle contractile function remains unclear and represents a challenging topic in the future because the circadian variation in muscle force is generally in phase with the circadian variation in body core temperature. It is hypothesized that the diurnal increase in core temperature could have a beneficial passive warm-up effect.

It is possible to shift the acrophase of the muscle power variation by a couple of hours following a few days by adapting sleep and meal schedules. Moreover, the use of another source of passive warm-up (e.g., a warm environment) seems to blunt the diurnal variation in muscle power. With long duration exercise, the thermal stress induced by physical exercise in a warm (and humid) environment should be higher in the evening, when the initial body temperatures are the highest.

Physical activities have to be considered for their effect on health. For example, cardiac events occur mainly between 06:00 - 12:00 h and a vigorous physical activity could be a trigger for them. Clinicians should advise at risk patients to avoid exercise at this time-of-day. Physical activity can also have some beneficial effects. For example, physical activity increases the amplitude of some circadian variations in elderly people allowing for the improvement both nocturnal sleep quality (i.e., less) and diurnal vigilance.

Chapter 9 - Recent burnout research has examined coaches and athletes collectively to determine the influence of coach behaviors on coach and athlete burnout. Results revealed a potential incongruity between decision-making behaviors and their influence on coach and athlete burnout. Therefore, the present study examined relationships between decision-making styles of coaches and burnout among coaches and athletes; gender influence on burnout was also examined. Collegiate swimmers and swimming coaches completed questionnaires assessing burnout and decision-making behaviors. Results revealed a significant relationship between athlete burnout and autocratic coaching behaviors. A significant inverse relationship emerged between athlete burnout and democratic behaviors. Significant main effects were found for democratic behaviors on exhaustion and depersonalization subscales; swimmers perceiving fewer democratic behaviors scored higher on these subscales. No significant relationships or gender differences were found with the coaches. Results suggest that coaches eliciting feedback from athletes could reduce the likelihood of burnout among those athletes without predisposing themselves.

In: Hot Topics in Sports and Athletics
Editor: Samuel R. Bakere, pp. 1-15

ISBN 978-1-60456-077-0

Chapter 1

Sports Advertising and Body Image

Dave Smith*[*]*, Caroline Wright, Natalie Ross and Sarah Warmington
University of Chester, Chester CH1 4BJ United Kingdom

Abstract

These studies examined the effects of sport-related advertising on body image. In Study 1, two hundred and twenty four collegiate females were categorised into regular exercisers and non-exercisers. In the pre-test and post-test (i.e., before and after exposure to advertising), each participant completed the Silhouette Measure of Body Image (SMBI; Stunkard, Sorenson and Schlusinger, 1983), the 9-item Social Physique Anxiety Scale (Martin, Rejeski, Leary, McAuley and Bane, 1997) and the Attitudes Towards Sport Advertisements (ATSA; adapted by Sabiston and Monroe, 2001, from Rabak-Wagner, Eickoff-Shemek and Kely-Vance, 1998), and the exercisers completed the 7-subscale Reasons for Exercise Inventory (Silberstein, Striegel-Moore, Timko and Rodin, 1988). They were then assigned to the model or product-related advertising condition. Participants were shown 15 sport-related advertisements either showing models (model condition) or workout shoes (product condition). Participants were given five minutes to view the advertisements, and then completed the questionnaires again. The results showed that the exercisers who were exposed to the model condition scored significantly ($p<.01$) higher on all measures in the post-test compared to the pre-test. The non-exercisers exposed to the model condition increased significantly ($p<.05$) on all measures from pre- to post-test but scored significantly ($p<.05$) lower on all post-test measures than the exerciser group. The product condition groups did not increase significantly on any measure ($p>.05$ in all cases). In Study 2, two hundred and forty nine sedentary undergraduates (126 males, 123 females) completed the SPAS, the SMBI and the ATSA. Following the pre-test, participants were shown 15 sport-related same-sex advertisements. Participants were given five minutes to view the advertisements, before completing the measures again. Group x test ANOVAs revealed that, in both the pre-test and the post-test, females scored significantly ($p<.05$) higher than males on the SMBI

* Correspondence concerning this article should be addressed to Dr Dave Smith, University of Chester, Parkgate Road, Chester, CH1 4BJ, UK.

and SPAS. The SMBI, SPAS and ATSA scores of the female participants, and the SPAS and ATSA scores of the males, increased significantly ($p<.05$) from pre- to post-test. Males' SMBI scores were higher in the post-test than the pre-test but the difference was not statistically significant ($p>.05$). These results show that the use of very fit and toned models in the advertising of sport-related products can have a detrimental effect upon body image of both males and females.

Keywords: *body image, sport, advertising.*

Current societal pressures for female attractiveness place a huge emphasis on the ideal of thinness, which is accepted by most women but impossible for the majority to attain (Tiggemann, 2004). The current sociocultural ideal for males emphasizes a larger, more muscular physique, with a well defined upper body (Pope and Gruber, 1997; Pope, Philips and Olivardia, 2000; Leit, Pope and Gray, 2001). Again, however, this 'ideal' is very different from the average male physique. This is unfortunate as Spitzer, Henderson and Zivian (1999) suggest that people with a large discrepancy between their body image and their bodily ideal tend to show negative attitudes towards their body and may engage in unhealthy behaviours, such as extreme low calorie diets or bulimic eating patterns in the case of females, or anabolic steroid use in males. Therefore, a comprehensive understanding of the factors affecting body image is important for those attempting to prevent or treat such behaviours. The aim of the studies presented in this chapter was to examine the influence of one factor that may exert a considerable influence on individuals' body dissatisfaction, that of sports advertising.

Body image is conceptualised as being malleable (Graham, Eich, Kephart and Peterson, 2000), meaning that it can be shaped or altered by various influences such as; media (Groesz, Levine and Murden, 2001), peers (Stice, Maxfield and Wells, 2003), and culture (Yang, Gray and Pope, 2005). Research has shown that these societal influences are capable of affecting body image perceptions in both males and females. However, Groesz et al. (2001, p.2) claim that the media, including advertisers, are the "loudest and most aggressive purveyors" of body image ideals, using them to sell and promote their products to target audiences.

Evans, Berman and Wellington (1997) describe advertising as something that is designed to inform and persuade potential customers. Advertisements are intended to have an initial impact on a targeted audience and are seen daily in magazines, on billboards, on television and on the Internet. Body image dissatisfaction among males and females is the result of social comparison against unrealistic body ideals, which are continually publicised through advertising and the mass media. Advertisements tend to emphasise extreme subgroups of 'thinness' for females and 'muscularity' for males (McDermott, 1996). These portray unattainable achievements in body weight, shape, and muscularity for the majority of people, which can lead to increased levels of body dissatisfaction (Lindeman, 1999). For example, a study by Hargreaves and Tiggemann (2004) focussed on adolescents who viewed television commercials containing images of 'thin' women, 'muscular' men or non-appearance commercials. They found that exposure to the commercials containing 'ideal' images led to increased body dissatisfaction amongst the female participants.

The commercials used by Hargreaves and Tiggemann (2004) appeared fairly typical examples of the way the media portray the 'ideal' body. For instance, Garner, Garfunkel, Schwartz and Thompson (1980) found that 69% of Playboy centrefolds and 60% of Miss America pageants were 15% or more below the average weight for their height and weight. Yamamiya, Cash, Melnyk, Posavac and Posavac (2005) suggest that the media force the thin ideal on to the consumers by encouraging them that they 'can' and 'should' be thin. They do this through educating them into how to obtain these thin ideals. For example, women's magazines often contain articles that describe methods for losing weight. Wiseman, Gray, Moismann and Aherns (1992) supported this and found from reviewing women's magazines over a 30-year period that there was a total increase in the number of articles relating to exercise and dieting. Stice, Schupak-Nemberg, Shaw and Stein (1994) found that the more a person was exposed to magazines and television during the previous month, the higher the levels of body dissatisfaction he or she reported. Stice et al. concluded from this that the media portray ideals that are unrealistic and cause females to have negative feelings towards their body. The 'thin,' 'muscular', ideals that are portrayed within the media may affect people's attitudes towards their body and lead to increased body dissatisfaction (Hart et al., 1989).

Historically, body dissatisfaction among females has attracted more research interest than that among males, partly because the research has indicated that women report higher levels of body dissatisfaction than men and place a greater value on losing weight. This is thought to contribute to their increased risk of developing an eating disorder (Grover, Keel and Mitchell, 2003; Garner et al., 1980). For example, Grover et al. (2003) found that normal weight women rated themselves heavier than normal weight males, despite there being no actual difference in body size. Furnham and Radley (1989) reported that slightly overweight males were more accepted by both males and females than slightly overweight females. These results suggest that there is a greater pressure for thinness and a narrower acceptability among females than males. Western culture may account for these differences due to the large emphasis they place on thinness as a female ideal of beauty (Garner et al., 1980; Striegel-Moore, Silberstein and Rodin, 1986; Furnham and Radley, 1989; Stice et al., 2003).

However, over the past few decades there has been increasing evidence of body image disorders in males (Holle, 2004; Leit, Gray and Pope, 2002). McCabe and Ricciardelli (2004) reviewed literature on male body image across the lifespan and found that college men were equally divided between wanting to lose weight and wanting to gain weight. They suggested that the discrepancy between the levels of body dissatisfaction among males and females was because studies relied on whether males wanted to lose weight and did not take into account whether males wanted to gain weight. From their review, they proposed that by questioning both dimensions in males, similar levels of body dissatisfaction would be demonstrated between males and females.

According to Holle (2004) there has been an increase in body dissatisfaction in males over recent decades. The results of his study showed that self-perceived overweight and underweight men reported less willingness to volunteer for activities that may involve the body being scrutinised by others than self-perceived normal weight men. A further finding was that an unwillingness to expose the upper torso was significantly associated with a higher fear of negative evaluation and increased social physique anxiety (Holle, 2004). This rise in body dissatisfaction might reflect the increased media attention paid to the muscular male ideal. Pope, Olivardia, Borowiecki and Cohane (2001) analysed advertisements in two American women's magazines from 1958-1998. They counted the number of males and females in each advert and calculated the state to which they were undressed. The findings indicated that from 1958-1998, the level of undressed females in advertisements remained at 20%, but the level of undressed males rose from 3%-35%. Leit et al. (2001) analysed Playgirl centrefolds over a 25-year period (1973-1997) and found that the male body ideal had become increasingly more muscular over the years (especially during the 1990's). Pope, Olivardia, Gruber, and Borowiecki (1999) supported these findings with the level of muscularity in action toys increasing to levels that are impossible to obtain in reality, even for professional bodybuilders consuming large doses of anabolic steroids. The trends that are found within these studies, such as increases in muscularity and increases in male exposure to magazines pose problems when viewed through Festinger's (1954) social comparison theory. This is because men are comparing themselves to unrealistic body images that cannot be achieved through natural methods and could lead to body dissatisfaction (Kimmel and Mahalik, 2004). Leit et al. (2002) supported this, finding that exposure to advertisements containing images of muscular male figures led to an increase in body dissatisfaction. Perceived pressure to adhere to these advertisements has resulted in some males suffering from body image concerns and indulging in pathological behaviours, such as excessive exercising, extreme dieting and steroid use, to achieve this sociocultural ideal (Lantz, Rhea and Mayhew, 2001).

Advertising in general has been shown to affect both males' and females' body image, but does sports advertising affect them in the same way? This is an important question, because the representations of the body used in sports advertising may be perceived by the general public as the standard to which their bodies would be compared in sport or exercise environments. This may affect the activities they choose to participate in and lead to avoidant behaviours, as they are worried about others evaluating their body in a negative way (Crawford and Eklund, 1994; Hart, Leary and Rejeski, 1989). Thus, as some sport psychologists have suggested (Crawford and Eklund, 1994; Hart et al., 1989; Lantz, Hardy and Ainsworth, 1997), individuals with such concerns are more likely to avoid exercise and sports settings where their body can be evaluated by others. Given such potential outcomes, particularly in the context of rising obesity levels and an increasingly sedentary lifestyle in the western world, the possible impact of sports advertising on body image is an important issue for investigation.

Recognising the importance of this issue, Sabiston and Munroe (2001) examined whether sports advertisements were led to increased social physique anxiety in female athletes. Social physique anxiety is a type of body image concern where individuals feel anxious regarding the prospect of others evaluating their physiques (Hart et al., 1989). In their study comparing the effect of exposure to model-only advertising and product-only advertising on social physique anxiety, Sabiston and Munroe found that, after female athletes were exposed to model-only advertising, their social physique anxiety increased, particularly in those who were initially low in social physique anxiety. They suggested that sports advertising could be associated with increased levels of social physique anxiety, but that more research was needed.

The aim of our studies was to build on these findings by examining the effects of sport-related advertising on social physique anxiety and body image disturbance in female and male exercisers and non-exercisers. We hypothesized that the body image disturbance scores of all groups would increase after exposure to model-related advertisments. In Study 1, which focused on comparing female exercisers and non-exercisers, we also hypothesized that increases in body image disturbance would be significantly greater in the exercisers, due to reports of a high incidence of body image disturbances in athletic populations (Petrie, 1993).

In Study 2, which focused on comparing males and females, we hypothesised that males' and females' body image would be disturbed to an equal degree following exposure to the advertising.

Study 1 Method

Participants

Two hundred and twenty four females between 18 and 25 years were divided into four groups: regular exercisers exposed to model-related advertising, non-exercisers exposed to model-related advertising, regular exercisers exposed to product-related advertising and non-exercisers exposed to product-related advertising. Regular exercisers were defined as those who reported participating in some form of purposeful exercise activity (e.g. running, aerobics, weight training) at least once per week. All participants provided written informed consent prior to participation.

Measures

Silhouette Measure of Body Image (SMBI; Stunkard, Sorenson and Schlusinger, 1983)

The SMBI was used to measure the cognitive modality of body image, an integral thought process in which one evaluates and gains a perception of one's bodily shape and size. It is a 9-point continuum of body figure diagrams, ranging from extremely thin to extremely overweight. Respondents rate their current and ideal body size, and scores are calculated by subtracting the 'ideal' figure rating from the 'current' figure rating. The SMBI has been validated as an anthropometric body size measure, with correlations between body weight and silhouette choice ranging from .65 to .84 for untrained observers and .85 to .92 for trained observers (Mueller, Joos and Schull, 1985). Cohn and Adler (1992) supported the concurrent validity of the scale by finding a strong relationship ($r = .76$) between SMBI scores and self-reported weight dissatisfaction. Also, the internal consistency of the scale is high ($\alpha = .92$; Lavine, Sweeney and Wagner, 1999).

Social Physique Anxiety Scale (SPAS; Martin, Rejeski, Leary, McAuley and Bane, 1997)

The SPAS was used to measure the affective component of body image. It is a 9-item, Likert-scored scale that measures the extent to which participants become anxious about others evaluating their physical appearance. Items include "Unattractive features of my figure make me feel nervous in certain social settings" and "When in a bathing suit, I often feel nervous about the shape of my body". The 9-item SPAS has demonstrated acceptable test-retest reliability ($\alpha = .82$) and internal consistency (Cronbach's $\alpha = .90$, Martin et al., 1997). Also, the construct validity of the 9-item scale has been supported by significant correlations between the SPAS and several related scales (Motl and Conroy, 2000).

Reasons for Exercise Inventory (Silberstein, Striegel-Moore, Timko and Rodin, 1988)

This is a 24-item, 7-subscale Likert-scored scale that evaluates motives for exercising. The subscales are weight control, health, fitness, improving body tone, improving physical attractiveness, mood enhancement and enjoyment. Respondents rate the importance of each motive on a scale of 1 (not at all important) to 7 (extremely important). For the purposes of this study we were only interested in the weight control and attractiveness subscales, as these are indicative of the behavioral modality of body image (Sabiston and Munroe, 2001). According to Silberstein et al. (1988), all subscales demonstrate acceptable internal consistency ($\alpha > .70$ in all cases except the attractiveness subscale, where $\alpha = .70$).

Attitudes Towards Sport Advertising Scale (ATSA; adapted by Sabiston and Monroe from Rabak-Wagener, Eickoff-Shemek and Kely-Vance, 1998)

The ATSA is an 11-item Likert-scored scale that measures beliefs and behaviours towards sport advertising. It is based upon Rabak-Wagener et al.'s Attitudes Towards Fashion advertising Scale, with the word "fashion" replaced by the word "sport" where appropriate. A total score is calculated from the 11 items to measure overall perception of body image (Rabak-Wagener et al., 1988). The higher the total score, the greater the body image disturbance. Rabak-Wagener et al. found the original scale to have a high test-retest reliability ($\alpha = .82$).

Procedure

Participants completed all the questionnaires and were then randomly assigned to the model or product-related advertising condition. On a separate occasion, participants were shown 15 exercise-related advertisements either showing female models (model-related condition) or running and workout shoes (product-related condition). The advertisements used were identical to those used by Sabiston and Monroe (2001). They were taken from popular sport and fitness magazines published in the US and Canada, including Shape, Fitness and Self. Each participant was given five minutes to view the advertisements, and then completed the questionnaires again.

Study 1 Results

Pre- and post-test means and standard deviations for the SMBI, SPAS, REI weight control, REI attractiveness and ATSA are shown in Figures 1 to 5 respectively. Group x test ANOVAs revealed significant effects for the SMBI for both test, $F(1,220) = 44.41$, $p<.001$, and group x test, $F(3, 220) = 24.28$, $p<.001$. This was also the case for the SPAS, $F(1,220) = 151.73$, $p<.001$ (test), $F(3,220) = 67.11$, $p<.001$ (group x test), REI weight control, $F(1,110) = 22.51$, $p<.001$ (test), $F(1,110) = 14.11$, $p<.001$ (group x test), REI attractiveness, $F(1,110) = 24.57$, $p<.001$ (test), $F(1,110) = 16.03$, $p<.001$ (group x test), and the ATSA, $F(1,220) = 121.66$, $p<.001$ (test), $F(3,220) = 34.96$, $p<.001$ (group x test). Tukey HSD tests revealed no significant between-group pre-test differences ($p>.05$ in all cases). The exercisers and non-exercisers who were exposed to the model-related condition scored significantly higher on all scales in the post-test compared to the pre-test ($p<.05$ in all cases). However, the non-exercisers scored significantly lower on all scales in the post-test than the exerciser group ($p<.05$ in all cases). The product-condition groups did not increase significantly on any scales in the post-test ($p>.05$ in all cases).

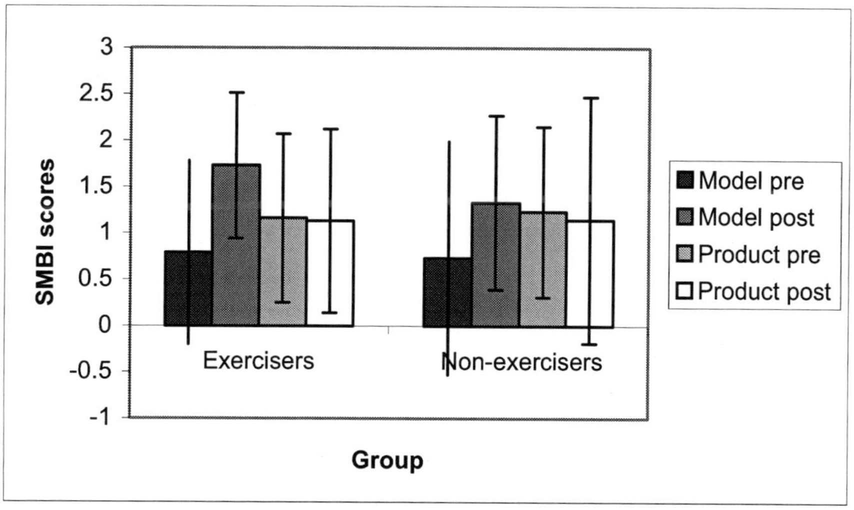

Figure 1. Mean and standard deviation pre- and post-test Silhouette Measure of Body Image scores for model and product conditions.

Study 2 Method

Participants and Measures

Two hundred and forty nine sedentary undergraduates (126 males, 123 females) between the ages of 18 and 26 were given the SPAS, the SMBI and the ATSA. As in Study 1, all participants provided written informed consent prior to participation.

Procedure

For the pre-test, participants completed all the questionnaires. On a separate occasion following the pre-test, participants were shown 15 exercise-related advertisements showing either female models (for the female participants) or male models (for the male participants). The female model advertisements were identical to those used in Study 1. The male model advertisements were taken from the following sports and fitness magazines: *Body Fitness*, *Exercise Protocol, MuscleMag* and *Swimrite*. Each participant was given five minutes to view the advertisements, and then completed the SMBI, SPAS and ATSA again.

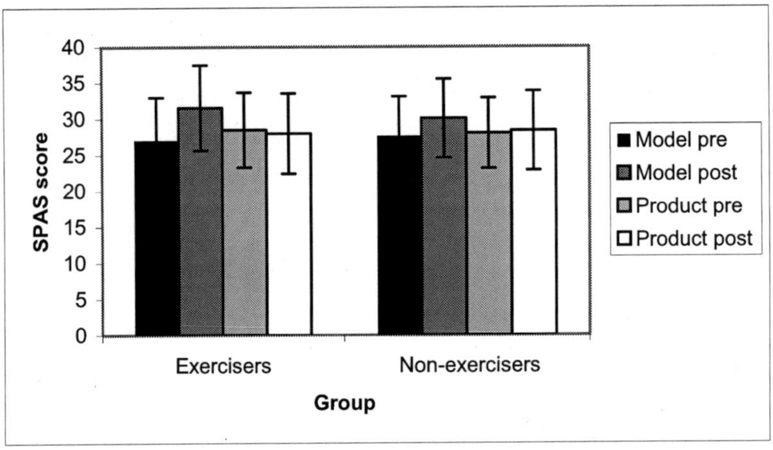

Figure 2. Mean and standard deviation pre- and post-test Social Physique Anxiety Scale scores for model and product conditions.

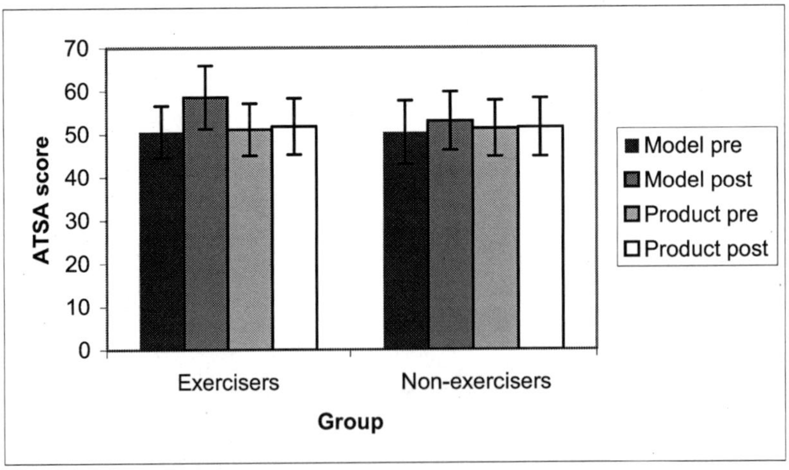

Figure 3. Mean and standard deviation pre- and post-test Attitudes towards Sports Advertising scores for model and product conditions.

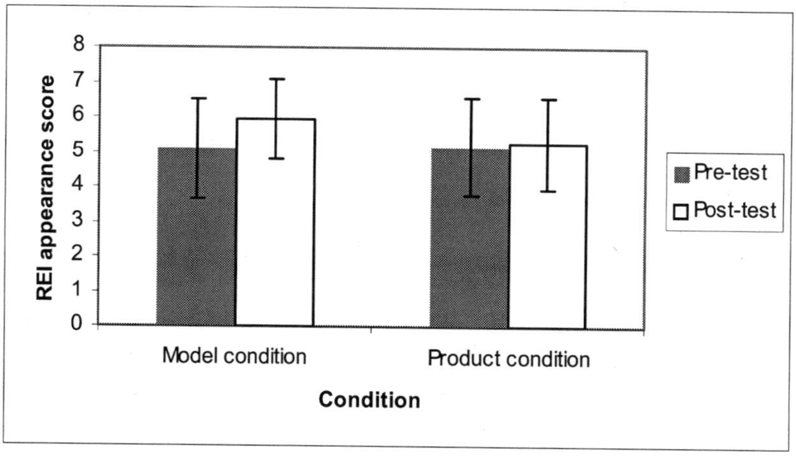

Figure 4. Mean and standard deviation pre- and post-test Reasons for Exercise Inventory appearance subscale scores for model and product conditions.

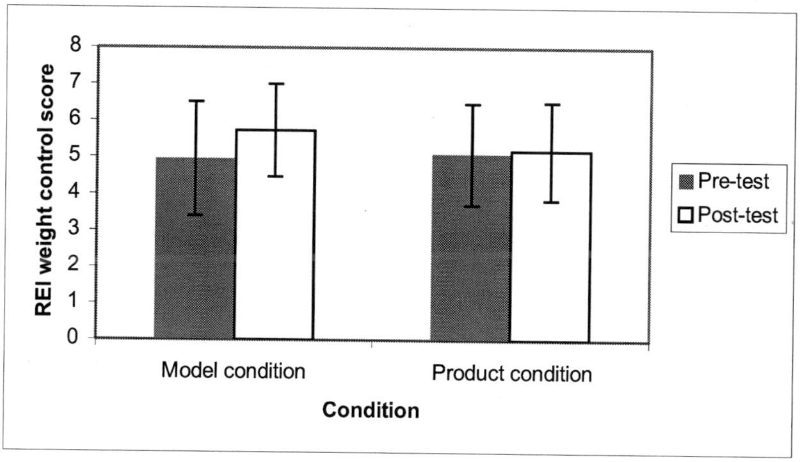

Figure 5. Mean and standard deviation pre- and post-test Reasons for Exercise Inventory weight control subscale scores for model and product conditions.

Study 2 Results

Pre- and post-test mean and standard deviation SMBI, SPAS and ATSA scores are shown in Figures 6 to 8 respectively. A group x test ANOVA for the SMBI revealed a significant effect for test, $F(1,247) = 49.99$, $p<.001$ and group x test, $F(1,247) = 13.83$, $p<.001$. In both the pre-test and the post-test, females scored significantly higher than males. The SMBI scores of the female participants increased significantly ($p<.05$) from pre- to post-test. In contrast, though males' SMBI scores were slightly higher in the post-test than the pre-test, the difference was not statistically significant ($p>.05$).

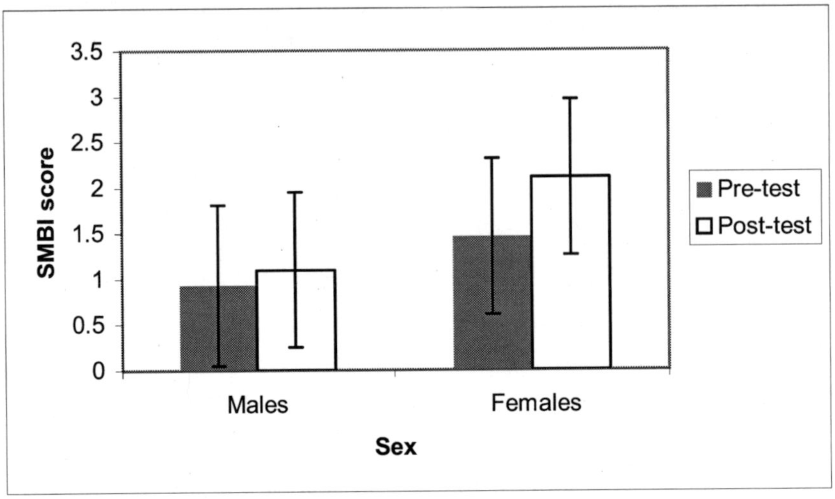

Figure 6. Mean and standard deviation pre- and post-test Silhouette Measure of Body Image scores for males and females.

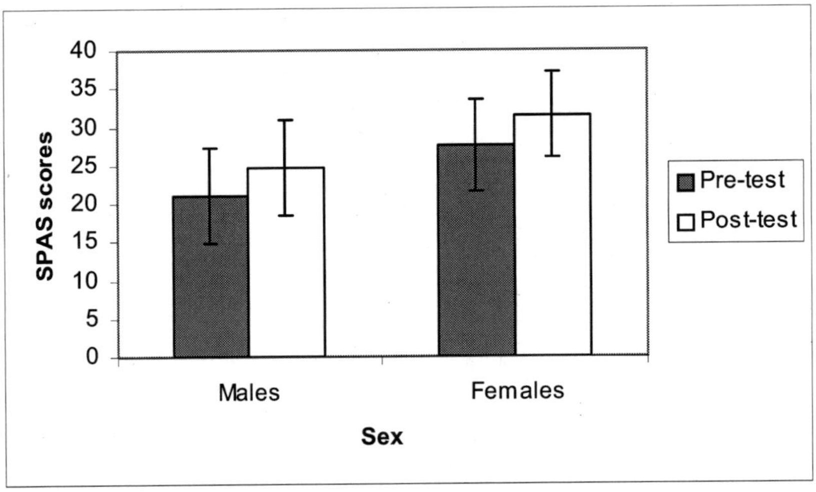

Figure 7. Mean and standard deviation pre- and post-test Social Physique Anxiety Scale scores for males and females.

A group x test ANOVA for the SPAS also revealed a significant for test, $F(1,247) = 410.25$, $p<.001$. However, there was no significant group x test effect, $F(1,247) = 1.06$, $p>.05$, and thus although SPAS scores increased from pre-test to post-test, there was no difference between the groups in the magnitude of the increases. This was also the case with the ATSA, with a significant effect for test. Similar results were found with the ATSA, with a significant effect for test, $F(1,247) = 224.25$, $p<.001$ but no significant group x test interaction, $F(1,247) = 1.23$, $p>.05$.

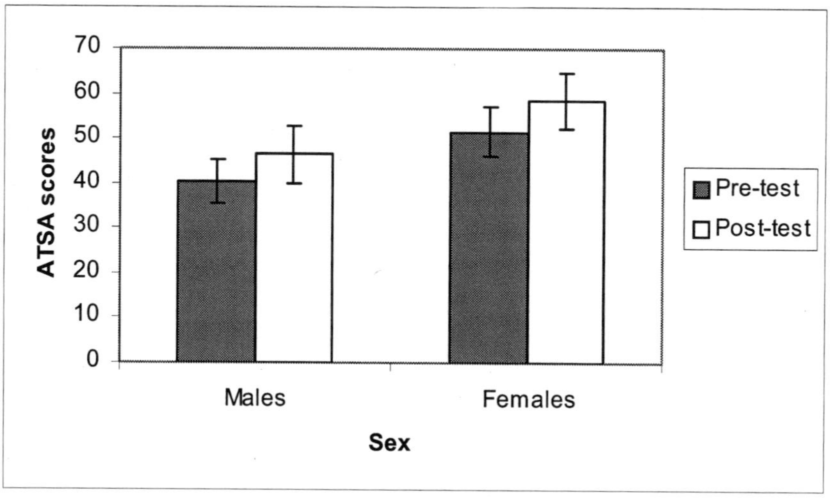

Figure 8. Mean and standard deviation pre- and post-test Attitudes Towards Sports Advertising scores for males and females.

Conclusion

The results of these studies concur with the conclusions of Sabiston and Munroe (2001), that the use of very fit and toned models in the advertising of exercise-related products can have a detrimental effect upon body image. All groups of participants exposed to model-related advertising in our two studies showed changes in SPAS and SBMI scores, and in three out of four cases these changes were statistically significant. In contrast, those participants viewing the product-related advertisements did not increase significantly in their SPAS or SBMI scores. Therefore, it is clearly not sports advertising per se, but rather the use of very slim, fit, healthy and attractive models in such advertising that leads to such body image disturbances. These results can be explained by Festinger's (1954) social comparison theory, which emphasises the importance of comparisons with social norms when individuals are evaluating themselves. It appears that the participants compared themselves to the 'ideal', slim, toned or muscular figures shown within the advertisements, which altered how they perceived and evaluated their bodies. The advertisements apparently instilled feelings of inadequacy about the participants' figures and provided an unrealistic standard for comparison. What is particularly noteworthy about this is that these changes in body image occurred after just a few minutes' exposure to the advertisements. Presumably, such increases in body image dissatisfaction will be small compared to the effects of the chronic exposure to such advertisements that individuals experience outside of the experimental setting. This assumption is supported by Stice et al.'s (1994) finding that the more people were exposed to magazines and television, the higher their levels of body dissatisfaction.

In Study 1, the body image of both exercisers and sedentary individuals was detrimentally affected, but the exercisers were affected to a significantly greater degree. As improving the attractiveness of one's body is a major motive for exercise, it appears reasonable to suggest that body attractiveness may be of greater concern to the exercising population. Therefore, they may be more affected by media images such as the ones used in this study, becoming more dissatisfied with their bodies as they begin to compare them with such unrealistic role models. This is very unfortunate, given the links between body dissatisfaction and eating disorders and pathogenic weight control methods.

Although the exercisers in Study 1 were affected more than the sedentary individuals, in one sense the results of the latter group are of even greater concern. That is, as poor body image and high social physique anxiety can make individuals less likely to want to exercise in front of others, the effect of exercise-related advertising on exercise participation and adherence may be very negative. This should be of concern not just to those involved in health and exercise promotion, but also to the advertisers themselves, who may be making a large proportion of their potential market less likely to exercise and, therefore, less likely to buy their products. Of course, the present studies did not actually examine the effect of these body image changes on intention to exercise. Therefore, researchers may wish to examine this by, for example, exposing sedentary individuals in the contemplation stage of exercise behaviour change to advertisements and examining the effect on their intention to exercise. It must be noted that despite the influential power of sport advertising, personality traits may also contribute to the likelihood of developing body image disturbances, and therefore this is also an area worthy of future research, to enable identification of individuals most at risk.

In Study 2, the detrimental effects of exercise-related advertising in sedentary females were again clearly demonstrated. There was also a significant increase for the males on the SPAS and ATSA, showing that the body image disturbance in males can also be increased by exposure to sports advertising. Therefore, our SPAS and ATSA findings show that this is not just a female problem, adding further support to the findings of Leit et al. (2002), who found that exposure to muscular male ideals resulted in males having a large discrepancy between their ideal muscularity and their perceived muscularity. However, our findings on the SMBI appear to contradict this, as the male SMBI scores did not increase significantly after exposure to the advertisements. We argue, however, that this finding may reflect the nature of the measure used (SMBI). This is because the SMBI does not clearly represent different levels of muscularity, just levels of thinness and fatness, and the figure drawings do not clearly show muscular definition. Therefore, future research should use a measure, such as that developed by Hildebrandt, Langenbucher and Schlundt (2004), which shows clear muscular dimensions on the figure drawings. This measure could successfully be used to examine whether males strive towards a more muscular, rather than a slimmer physique.

These findings have some important practical implications. Clearly, sport-related advertising in its typical current form, with very thin female models and very muscular male models, has a detrimental effect on people's body image. To reduce this effect, the use of a mixture of body shapes (of average weight) within advertising, is recommended. Such a change would not only be useful in producing more realistic and psychologically healthy body shape ideals, but may also be useful for the advertisers, allowing more people to relate to the advertisements, hence increasing the target audience. Of particular relevance to sports advertising, more average, realistic body images should also be used in the advertising of sports and fitness facilities and products, as this could encourage sedentary individuals to use such facilities and buy such products. This would produce benefits for both those advertising such facilities and products, and for public health.

References

Cohn, L. D., and Alder, N. E. (1992). Female and male perceptions of ideal body shapes. *Psychology of Women Quarterly, 16*, 69-79.

Crawford, S., and Eklund, R. (1994). Social Physique Anxiety, Reasons for exercise and attitudes towards exercise settings. *Journal of Sport and Exercise Psychology, 16*, 70-82.

Evans, J, R., Berman, B., and Wellington, W. J. (1997). *Marketing.* Scarborough, Prentice Hall Canada Inc.

Festinger, L. (1954). A theory of social comparison processes. *Human Relations, 7*, 117-140.

Furnham, A., and Radley, S. (1989). Sex differences in the perception of male and female body shapes. *Personality and Individual Differences, 10*, 653-662.

Garner, D. M., Garfinkel, D., Schwartz, D., and Thompson, M. (1980). Cultural expectations of thinness in women. *Psychology Reports, 47*, 483-491.

Graham, M. A., Eich, C., Kephart, B., and Peterson, D. (2000). Relationship among body image, sex, and popularity of high school students. *Perceptual and Motor Skills, 90*, 1187-1193.

Groesz, L. M., Levine, M. P., and Murnen, S. K. (2001). The Effect of Experimental Presentation of Thin Media Images on Body Satisfaction: A Meta-Analytic Review. *International Journal of Eating Disorders, 31 (1)*, 1-16.

Grover, V. P., Keel, P. K., and Mitchell, J. P. (2003). Gender Differences In Implicit Weight Identity. *International Journal of Eating Disorders, 34 (1)*, 125-135.

Hargreaves, D. A., and Tiggemann, M. (2004). Idealized media images and adolescent body image: 'comparing boys and girls'. *Body Image, 1*, 351-361.

Hart, E. A., Leary, M. R., and Rejeski, W. J. (1989) The measurement of social physique anxiety. *Journal of Sport and Exercise Psychology,11*, 94-104.

Hildebrandt, T., Langenbucher, J., and Schlundt, D.G. (2004). Muscularity concerns among men: development of perceptual and attitudinal measures. *Body Image: An International Journal of Research, 1*, 169–81.

Holle, C. (2004). Male Body Image: Self-Perceived Weight Status and Avoidance of Body Exposure. *Perceptual and Motor Skills, 99 (3)*, 853-860.

Kimmel, S. B., and Mahalik, J. R. (2004). Measuring masculine body ideal distress: development of a measure. *International Journal of Mens Health, 3*, 1-11.

Lantz, C. D., Hardy, C. J., and Ainsworth, B. E. (1997). Social Physique Anxiety and perceived exercise behaviour. *Journal of Sport Behaviour, 20*, 83-93.

Lantz, C. D., Rhea, D. J., and Mayhew, J. L. (2001). The drive for size: a psycho behavioural model of muscle dysmorphia. *International Sports Journal, 5 (1)*, 71-86.

Lavine, H., Sweeney, D., and Wagner, S. H. (1999). Depicting women as sex objects in television advertising: Effects on body dissatisfaction. *Personality and Social Psychology Bulletin, 25*, 1049-1058.

Leit, R. A., Gray, J. J., and Pope, Jr., H. G. (2002). The Media's Representation of the Ideal Male Body: A Cause for Muscle Dysmorphia?. *International Journal of Eating Disorders, 31(3)*, 334-338.

Leit, R. A., Pope, Jr., H. G., and Gray, J. J. (2001). Cultural expectations of muscularity in men: The evolution of Playgirl centerfolds. *International Journal of Eating Disorders, 29*, 90–93.

Lindeman, A. K. (1999). Quest for ideal weight: Costs and consequences. *Medicine Science In Sports and Exercise, 31*, 1135-1140.

Martin, K. A., Rejeski, W. J., Leary, M. R., McAuley, E., and Bane, S. (1997). Is the Social Physique Anxiety Scale Really Multidimensional? Conceptual and Statistical Arguments for a Unidimensional Model. *Journal of Sport and Exercise Psychology, 19*, 359-367.

McCabe, M. P., and Ricciardelli, L. A. (2004). Body image dissatisfaction among males across the lifespan: A review of past literature. *Journal of Psychosomatic Research, 56 (6)*, 675-685.

McDermott, L. (1996). Toward a feminist understanding of physicality within the context of women's physically active and sporting lives. *Sociology of Sport Journal, 13, 1*, 1230.

Motl, R., and Conroy, D. E. (2000). Validity and factorial invariance of the Social Physique Anxiety Scale. *Medicine and Science in Sports and Exercise, 32*, 1007-1017.

Mueller, W. H., Joos, S. K., and Schull, W. J. (1985). Alternative measurements of obesity: Accuracy of body silhouettes and reported weights and heights in a Mexican/American sample. *International Journal of Obesity, 9*, 193-200.

Petrie, T. (1993). Disordered eating in female collegiate gymnasts: Prevalence and personality/attitudinal correlates. *Journal of Sport and Exercise Psychology, 15*, 424-436.

Pope, H. G. Jr., and Gruber, A. J. (1997). Muscle dysmorphia: An underrecognised form of body dysmorphic disorder. *Psychosomatics, 38*, 548-557.

Pope, H. G. Jr., Philips, K. A., and Olivardia, R. (2000). *The Adonis complex: The secret crisis of male body obsession.* New York: Free Press.

Rabak-Wagener, J., Eickoff-Shemeck, J., and Kelly-Vance, L. (1998). The effect of media analysis on attitudes and behaviors regarding body image among college students. *Journal of American College Health, 47 (1)* 29-37.

Sabiston, C. M., and Munroe, K.J. (2001). *The Effect of Sport and Fitness Advertising on Social Physique Anxiety among Females.* Proceedings of the annual meeting of the Association for the Advancement of Applied Sport Psychology. Denton, Texas: RonJon Publishing.

Silberstein, L. R., Striegel-Moore, R. H., Timko, C., and Rodin, J. (1988). Behavioural and psychological implications of body attractiveness for women. *Sex Roles, 14*, 519-532.

Spitzer, B. L., Henderson, K. A., and Zivian, M. T. (1999). Gender differences in population versus media body sizes: A comparison over four decades. *Sex Roles, 40*, 545–565.

Stice, E., Maxfield, J., and Wells, T. (2003). Adverse effects of social pressure to be thin on young women: An experimental investigation of the effects of "fat talk". *International Journal of Eating Disorders, 34 (1)*, 109-116.

Stice, E., Schupak-Nemberg, E., Shaw, H. E., and Stein, R. I. (1994). Relation of the media exposure to eating disorder symptomatology: An examination of mediating mechanisms. *Journal of Abnormal Psychology, 103*, 836-840.

Striegal-Moore, R., Silberstein, L. and Rodin, J. (1986). Toward an understanding of risk factors for Bulimia. *American Psychologist, 41, 3*, 246-263.

Stunkard, A., Sorensen, T., and Schlsinger, F. (1983). Use of the Danish Adoption Register for the study of obesity and thinness. In S. Kety (Ed.), *The genetics of neurological and psychiatric disorders* (pp.115-120). New York: Raven Press.

Tiggemann, M. (2004). Body image across the adult lifespan: stability and change. *Body Image, 1*, 29-41.

Wiseman, C. V., Gray, J. J., Moismann, J. E., and Aherns, A. H. (1992). Cultural expectations of thinness in women: an update. *International Journal of Eating Disorders, 11*, 85-89.

Yamamiya, Y., Cash, T. F., Melnyk, S. E., Posavac, H. D., and Posavac, S. S. (2005). Women's exposure to thin-and-beautiful media images: Body image effects of media-ideal internalization and impact-reduction interventions. *Body Image*, *2*, 74-80.

Yang, C-F. J., Gray, P., and Pope, Jr., H. G. (2005). Male Body Image in Taiwan Versus the West: Yanggang Zhiqi Meets the Adonis Complex. *The American Journal of Psychiatry, 162 (2)*, 263-269.

In: Hot Topics in Sports and Athletics
Editor: Samuel R. Bakere, pp. 17-50

ISBN 978-1-60456-077-0

Chapter 2

Eating Disorders in Athletes: A Review of the Literature

Kristin L. Cobb
Department of Health Research and Policy
Stanford University Medical Center, Stanford, CA 94305, USA

Abstract

Athletes are at increased risk for eating disorders (ED). Eating disorders in athletes may have severe physical and mental consequences, including failure to attain peak bone mass, low-trauma fractures and stress fractures, vertebral instability and curvature, prolonged psychological difficulties with weight and food, and even death. The high prevalence and unique nature of ED in athletes have led researchers to describe athlete-specific syndromes, including anorexia athletica and the female athlete triad of disordered eating, menstrual irregularity, and osteopenia/osteoporosis. Eating disorders in athletes have distinct etiologies and require specialized approaches to diagnosis, prevention, and treatment. Research on ED in athletes has increased dramatically in the past two decades, following the rapid increase in women's participation in athletics; however, many gaps remain in our understanding. Participation in weight-dependent sports may also account for a considerable proportion of ED in men, but male athletes have not been well studied. This chapter will critically review the latest research on ED in athletes, including: (1) issues in the measurement of ED, including the female athlete triad; (2) sport-and gender-specific prevalences; (3) risk and protective factors; (4) short and long-term sequelae; (5) prevention strategies; and (6) treatment strategies, including a review of pharmacologic agents to prevent or treat osteopenia and osteoporosis. This chapter will identify gaps in the current research and recommend directions for future research.

Introduction

Early work on ED in athletes focused on anorexia nervosa (AN) and bulimia nervosa (BN) in ballet dancers [1-4]. Early reports focused on the difficulty in distinguishing the naturally thin or normal dieting ballerina from the anorectic ballerina [2-3]. Maloney (1983) says that all ballet dancers have a justifiable interest in achieving an "ethereal" look, and comments [2]:

> Drawing the line between normal dieting and anorexia nervosa is especially crucial for physicians, dance instructors, choreographers, administrators, and dancers themselves. All ballet dancers are weight conscious, and most have dieted to control their weight. Some dancers utilize stimulants or laxatives and even vomit to keep trim. p. 550.

Maloney suggests that non-anorectic dancers who lose a significant amount of weight may demonstrate bizarre food behaviors and emotions secondary to starvation—including intense preoccupation with food, hoarding food, stealing, gorging, and social isolation—yet not meet the criteria for Diagnostic and Statistical Manual of Mental Disorders (DSM-III) diagnosis of AN or BN [5], for example, if they lack an intense fear of getting fat or distorted body image.

Szmukler et al. (1985) similarly remark that the high level of disturbances of weight, worries about weight, and menstrual irregularities in a top-ranked ballet school make it difficult to pick out the eating disorder cases from the "background noise" [3]. Moreover, the authors suggest that even when a diagnosis of AN is made in this population, it means something different than the same diagnosis outside of the subculture of ballet:

> When 'symptoms' are very common in a population which nonetheless seems to be functioning well socially, and in this case functioning at a very high level physically as well, then caution must be exercised in the significance which is attributed to them. p. 181.

Taken together, these two early reports paint an overly romanticized picture of eating pathology in ballet—as a transient and generally appropriate adaptation to the demands of an extraordinary pursuit. In this idealized picture, when a dancer crosses the fine line from normal weight concerns to diagnosable AN or BN, intervention is necessary, but prospects for recovery are good.

In the past two decades, research has shed considerable light on these early exploratory reports. We now believe that abusing laxatives, vomiting, or starving to achieve the ethereal look of near emaciation—even transiently—can have devastating long-term consequences. Athletes who do not meet the strict diagnostic criteria for AN or BN may still have serious eating problems (disordered eating) that are worthy of concern. For example, disordered eating can lead to menstrual irregularity and irreversible bone loss (the female athlete triad) [6-7]. Furthermore, an athlete who has developed the specific psychopathologies of AN or BN should be considered as serious a case as a non-athlete with clinical ED.

Eating pathology in athletes provides unique challenges for researchers and clinicians. Athletes face unique risk factors for the development of disordered eating by virtue of their sport. They may more easily hide disordered eating against the "background noise" of their sport and may use success in sport to deny or justify their condition. ED in athletes deserves separate consideration within the larger body of research on ED in general.

Case Report 1

Zanker et al. (2004) reported a prolonged case of female athlete triad in an elite distance runner [8]. The woman began running at 10 years old, and began restricting her caloric, fat, and carbohydrate intake at 11 years old (pre-menarche) to improve her running times. A successful runner, she averted medical attention for 13 years despite a low body fat, low body mass index (BMI), primary amenorrhea and multiple tibial and metatarsal stress fractures. She was finally referred to the report's authors at age 24.8 years, when her repeated stress fractures led to a suspicion of osteoporosis. At presentation, she was running up to 60 miles per week and also cycling and swimming. Her body mass index (BMI) was 16.3 kg/m^2 (45.1 kg, 166 cm) and her body fat was 8.3%. She had never menstruated. Dual-energy X-ray Absorptiometry (DXA) evaluation revealed osteoporosis at the hip and osteopenia at the spine. She was diagnosed with female athlete triad, advised to increase her energy intake, and prescribed oral contraceptives—which she took to start her menstrual cycle. The authors regularly evaluated the young woman from ages 24.8 to 36.9 years, including taking yearly bone density measurements. The patient stopped running at age 25.2 years because of stress fractures, but continued to bike 70-80 miles per week and swim 5-6 miles per week; she continued to lose weight, reducing her BMI to 15.0 kg/m^2 and her body fat to less than 4% by the time she was 29.8 years old. During this time, her bone density decreased even further and she suffered multiple osteoporotic fractures of the ribs and pelvis. At this point, she was no longer under the pressure to be thin for running, she was aware that her restrictive eating behaviors had led to symptomatic osteoporosis, and she was aware that her bone density was continuing to plummet, yet she persisted in her disordered eating behavior.

Then at age 33.5 years, after 22 years of following a restricted diet and exercising excessively, and nearly nine years after she learned of the severe consequences of her behaviors, she made a decision to gain weight. At last report (age 36.9 years), her BMI was 17.6 kg/m^2, her body fat was 11.8%, and her BMD had increased from its lowest point, but she still had osteoporosis at the hip and osteopenia at the spine. It is unclear if continued weight gains will result in continued increases in BMD. Even if she continues to gain weight, it is unlikely that her BMD will ever return to normal levels for her age.

Her case illustrates the serious nature of trying to achieve a waiflike body type for sport. Though the patient initiated these behaviors in what might be seen as a justified adaptation to the demands her sport—at which she excelled—it is readily apparent that her behaviors were not benign. Her disordered eating persisted for 22 years, long after running competition ceased; she suffered multiple lower limb stress fractures, and osteoporotic fractures of the ribs and pelvis; at 36.9 years, she has frank osteoporosis and continued psychological difficulty with weight and food. One can speculate that if she was not a successful distance runner, her visible low weight and low body fat might have brought her to the attention of an eating disorder specialist earlier in the course of her disease. As it was, she evaded medical attention for 13 years before anyone was alarmed enough to send her for osteoporosis testing. Not all cases of disordered eating in athletes become this extreme, but the potential for substantial harm should be recognized.

Definitions and Diagnostic Criteria

Disordered eating in athletes is best conceptualized as a spectrum: from mildly abnormal concerns about weight and food coupled with occasional pathogenic eating behaviors to clinically significant partial syndromes not quite meeting the diagnostic criteria for AN or BN to full blown eating disorders [7,9]. Where we choose to focus along this spectrum determines how we quantify prevalence, diagnose disordered eating/eating disorders in athletes, and shape treatment and prevention strategies. Indeed, many of the discrepancies in the literature on ED in athletes can be explained by differences in this choice of where to draw the line between "healthy" and "disordered." This chapter will focus on athletes meeting the DSM-IV requirements for anorexia nervosa (AN), bulimia nervosa (BN), and eating disorders not otherwise specified (EDNOS) [10], and also on athletes fitting the profile of the female athlete triad [6-7].

Anorexia Nervosa

Anorexia nervosa is characterized by a refusal to maintain body weight above 85% of expected weight for age and height, an intense fear of becoming fat, a distorted body image, and amenorrhea, i.e. the absence of at least 3 consecutive menstrual cycles [10].

Bulimia Nervosa

Bulimia nervosa is characterized by recurrent episodes of binge eating (rapid consumption of a large amount of food) and purging, either through vomiting, laxatives, diuretics, compensatory fasting, or excessive exercise. The binge and purge behavior occurs at least twice a week for 3 months. Self-evaluation is unduly influenced by body shape and weight [10].

Eating Disorders not Otherwise Specified

Eating disorders not otherwise specified are diagnosed in women who meet several, but not all, of the criteria of AN and BN, for example, a woman who binges and vomits weekly but not twice weekly. EDNOS have also been called "subclinical" eating disorders or "partial syndromes." Sundgot-Borgen and Torstveit (1993) gave specific diagnostic criteria for anorexia athletica—a subclinical variant of AN described in athletes [11]. Anorexia athletica will be considered as a variant of EDNOS here.

Female Athlete Triad

The female athlete triad is defined along a continuum, requiring a combination of: some degree of inadequate eating (in the extreme, a diagnosable eating disorder), some form of menstrual disorder (in the extreme, amenorrhea), and some degree of skeletal demineralization (in the extreme, osteopororsis) [12]. An energy deficit—often secondary to intentional disordered eating—is recognized as the initiating and causative factor of the triad [12-20]; therefore, from an eating disorder perspective, the triad can be conceptualized as any restrictive disordered eating that is severe enough to cause menstrual irregularity and either bone loss or bone deficits due to insufficient skeletal growth. Diagnosis requires a bone density test to evaluate skeletal mineralization.

Measurement Issues in Research

Because disordered eating encompasses a spectrum of behaviors and attitudes, disordered eating may be measured on a quantitative scale, for example, frequency of self-induced vomiting or score on a standardized eating disorder questionnaire. The two most widely used questionnaires are the Eating Attitudes Test (EAT) and the Eating Disorder Inventory (EDI) [21-24]. Quantitative measures allow comparisons between groups, but cannot be used to estimate prevalence of ED in athletes. To estimate prevalence, researchers have attempted to divide athletes into four groups: (1) normal diet and weight concerns, (2) "at-risk" for ED, (3) ENDOS (including subclinical and partial syndromes), and (4) full-blown AN or BN. While there are clear criteria for the diagnosis of AN and BN, the EDNOS and at-risk categories are less well defined, and researchers may differ widely on *what* they are trying to measure, accounting for many of the discrepancies in the literature.

Many researchers have used cut-off scores on a standardized eating disorder screening test to classify athletes as "at-risk" for EDNOS, AN, or BN, including ≥30 on the EAT-40, ≥20 on the EAT-26, or ≥14 on the EDI drive for thinness subscale [22,24]. Other researchers have classified athletes as at-risk if they report pathogenic eating behaviors, such as self-induced vomiting or laxative abuse, or specific physiologic features. The at-risk category is often difficult to interpret because criteria may not be sufficiently specific for ED. For example, a large study of NCAA Division I sports teams classified female athletes as at-risk if they had a BMI of less than 20kg/m^2 [25], well within the healthy range for women; this criterion identified 31% of women as at-risk, but the usefulness of this classification is questionable. It is unclear what percentage of at-risk athletes have EDNOS, AN, BN, or female athlete triad, or what percentage go on to develop these conditions in the future.

Studies should aim to identify cases of AN, BN, EDNOS, and/or female athlete triad. The structured clinical interview is the gold standard for diagnosing AN, BN, and EDNOS. Researchers also use diagnostic questionnaires, such as the Eating Disorder Examination-Questionnaire (EDE-Q) [26], to identify athletes with AN, BN, and EDNOS by self-report. Written questionnaires have higher misclassification rates, but are faster, easier, and cheaper to administer than the clinical interview. Two-staged designs combine the ease of self-report questionnaires with the accuracy of the clinical interview: in the first stage, at-risk athletes are identified from a larger pool by means of a screening questionnaire; in the second stage, only at-risk athletes and controls are interviewed to confirm diagnoses [11,27]. Two-stage designs increase the specificity of diagnosis (reduce false positives), but do not improve the sensitivity; false negatives on the screening questionnaire will not be interviewed.

Underreporting is a major concern. Athletes may deny that they have a problem, or may deliberately lie to avoid detection [28]. Anorectics typically score low on self-report screens for ED despite being obviously emaciated [29,30]. In one study of athletes, none of 87 respondents had evidence of ED on the EAT questionnaire, yet 16 (18%) entered treatment for ED within 2 years [13]. O'Connor, Lewis, and Kirchner (1995) cleverly asked college gymnasts to fake their answers on the EDI questionnaire, and identified a common "faking" profile [31]. In a second sample, 12% exhibited the faking profile, suggesting a significant proportion of athletes—probably the ones who feel they have something to hide—lie on written ED questionnaires [31].

Assuring athletes of anonymity and administering questionnaires and interviews without involving coaches may help minimize faking [11,27]. Some researchers have also suggested the use of more objective, physiologic measures of ED to minimize under-detection due to faking [29,32]. Stice, Telch, and Rizvi (2000) used BMI$<$17.5 kg/m^2 and amenorrhea of at least 3 months duration as sufficient criteria to identify cases of AN [29]. Black et al. (2003) suggested that athletic trainers could use a combination of physiological measures, such as BMI and diastolic blood pressure after standing up from sitting, to screen for ED in athletes during the pre-participation physical [32].

Even if athletes are willing to answer truthfully, athletes may have a different ED profile than non-athletes, requiring specialized screening and diagnostic tools. Questions about body dissatisfaction, body image distortion, and bingeing may not reliably distinguish between athletes with ED and athletes without ED. Athletes with ED may not present with distorted body image or body dissatisfaction [33-38]. Byrne and McLean (2002) found that athletes with ED did not score higher on body dissatisfaction than non-athlete controls [37]. They suggest that some athletes may adopt disordered eating practices while maintaining a realistic sense of their thin body size. Behaviors mimicking binge eating may be common in athletes without ED. Sundgot-Borgen and Torstveit [11,27] have found that athletes over-report bingeing, as binge-level quantities of food may be necessary for an athlete who is expending large amounts of energy. For example, swimmer Michael Phelps, 6-time gold medalist in the 2004 Summer Olympics, reportedly eats two egg-and-cheese sandwiches, a bowl of grits, a large omelet and a tall stack of chocolate chip pancakes just for breakfast. For a non-athlete this would be a binge, but for Phelps it is necessary fuel. Though some researchers have designed questionnaires or physiologic measures to specifically screen for ED in athletes [32,39-40], these have not been widely used or standardized. Researchers should collaborate on the development of standardized screening questionnaires for the detection of ED in athletes.

Elite athletes may also have a different ED profile than non-elite athletes. Hopkinson and Lock (2004) suggested that non-elite athletes have more of the typical psychological features of ED, whereas elite athletes have more of the typical physiological features [41]. Non-elite athletes with ED may be actively trying to achieve the body type of their elite counterparts, resulting in psychological stress and body dissatisfaction, whereas elite athletes with ED may have already attained a dangerously low weight (and accompanying amenorrhea) and may be relatively pleased with their overly thin bodies.

The optimal screening tool for ED combines questions about psychology (feelings and attitudes toward weight, food, body size and shape) and questions about physiology (weight, menstruation). Women answer truthfully and accurately to questions about menstruation, and irregular menstruation may be a marker for ED. Recent studies confirm that caloric imbalance (ie, insufficient energy intake for energy expended) rather than body composition, stress, or exercise, is the main cause of menstrual disturbances in female athletes [15-20]. Amenorrhea also may precede weight loss in women with ED. Thus, a two-stage design that sends both women with high weight and food concerns and women with menstrual irregularity to a second-stage clinical interview may have higher sensitivity for ED in athletes than a screening tool that only asks about disordered eating. In identifying cases of female athlete triad, menstrual irregularity alone could be used to identify at-risk athletes, who could then be evaluated clinically for disordered eating and low bone density.

Prevalence

Numerous studies have examined prevalence of disordered eating in athletes in a variety of sports. For reviews see: Byrne and McLean (2001) [42] and Smolak, Murnen, and Ruble (2000) [35]. Data on the prevalence of disordered eating and ED in athletes are contradictory. Studies generally agree that athletes have a higher frequency of disordered eating than non-athletes, particularly in sports emphasizing leanness or a low body weight, and that female athletes have more disordered eating than male athletes. However, some studies have failed to find higher rates of eating problems in athletes, or have found lower rates. Some studies have raised the possibility that non-elite female athletes may be protected from risk of ED [35].

Discrepancies in results are due in large part to the heterogeneity of the populations under study [35]—with respect to sport type, age, gender, competitive levels (elite, varsity, recreational, etc.), and geographical region. Studies also vary in *what* aspect of disordered eating they are measuring (see measurement, above) and in their quality and sample size. All prevalence studies should use a non-athletic control group to estimate baseline levels of disordered eating—as it's being defined in a given study—in the region and age group of the target population. Studies should also report age, gender, and sport-specific rates as possible to facilitate comparisons across studies. Attempts should be made to standardize definitions and measurement of disordered eating in athletes and to measure prevalence of EDNOS, AN, BN, and female athlete triad, rather than prevalence of athletes "at-risk" (see measurement above).

Sundgot-Borgen (1993, 2004) and Torstveit (2004) [11,27] and Byrne and McLean (2002) [37] have produced the most valid and reliable estimates of ED prevalence in elite male and female athletes to date (Table 1). Sundgot-Borgen and Torstveit used an elegant two-stage design, where nearly every elite Norwegian athlete (and a sample of non-athletic controls) was screened for ED by the EDI questionnaire and all athletes (and controls) identified as at-risk were evaluated by clinical interview to diagnose AN, BN, and EDNOS.

Female athletes were studied in 1990 and again in 1997 in several categories of sport. Rates of ED are remarkably consistent, with small increases in ED seen in all sports classes and in controls from 1990 to 1997 (Table 1). These studies convincingly demonstrate that, with the exception of athletes in power sports (throwing and sprints), all groups of elite male and female athletes have higher rates of AN, BN, and ENDOS than male and female controls, respectively; prevalence of ED is highest in sports in which low weight is a requirement or advantage, including anti-gravitation (men only), aesthetic (women only), weight-class, and endurance sports. Byrne and McLean interviewed 263 elite Australian athletes in 6 "thin-build" sports and 4 "normal-build" sports and 263 matched, non-athletic controls and found similar results for weight-dependent sports: elite male and female athletes in thin-build sports have higher rates of AN, BN, and ENDOS than controls (Table 1). For the normal-build sports, however, rates of ED were only moderately elevated in female athletes, and were not increased in male athletes. The discrepancies between the Norwegian and Australian studies may reflect differences in sports studied, in groupings of sports, and in sample size.

These studies definitively demonstrate a higher prevalence of ED in elite athletes in sports in which lower weight is an advantage or a requirement, and even in some sports where weight is a less critical factor. However, future studies are needed to determine the prevalence of ED in non-elite athletes, the prevalence of ED in individual high-risk sports, such as running and gymnastics, and the prevalence of female athlete triad.

This chapter will review the literature on prevalence of ED in female and male athletes and of female athlete triad, including historical aspects, sports-specific rates, discrepancies in the literature, and findings in non-elite athletes.

Female Athletes

Many studies in the literature continue to cite a range of 15%-62% for the prevalence of disordered eating in female athletes. Interestingly, these figures date back to a series of studies conducted by Rosen et al. in the mid-1980's [43-45] that found 15% of 487 young competitive swimmers [44] and 62% of 42 college gymnasts [45] practiced at least one pathogenic weight-control behavior, including using vomiting, diuretics, diet pills, or laxatives daily for at least one month. While these are alarming numbers and were provocative studies, they do not give reliable estimates of the true prevalence of disordered eating or eating disorders in female athletes. The studies were primarily descriptive, lacked a control group, measured at-risk behaviors rather than ED, and are now nearly twenty years out-dated.

In the past two decades, many controlled studies have examined whether female athletes have a higher rate of at-risk eating behaviors and attitudes than non-athletes, with conflicting results. Higher rates of weight and diet concerns have been found in selected populations of ballet dancers [4,46-50], distance runners [51], swimmers [52], lightweight rowers [53-54], gymnasts [55], and rhythmic gymnasts [56] compared with non-athletic controls or athletes in other sports. However, some studies have found no increase in risk or a decrease in risk of eating problems in runners [53,57-58], gymnasts [52], or mixed groups of college athletes [47,59].

Table 1. Estimated prevalence of eating disorders (ED), including anorexia and bulimia nervosa and eating disorders not otherwise specified, in elite female athletes and controls in Norway in 1990† and 1997‡ and in Australia§

Sports Groupings and Numbers*	Technical	Endurance	Aesthetic	Weight class	Anti-gravitation Sports**	Ball games	Power	Overall	Controls
	Alpine skiing Bowling Golf High jump Horseback riding Long jump Rifle Shooting Sailing Sky diving 1990, n=98 1997, n=72 Men, n=97	Biathlon X-C skiing Cycling Dog racing Distance running Orienteering Race walking Rowing Speed skating Swimming 1993, n=119 1997, n=102 Men, n=149	Diving Figure skating **Gymnastics** Rhythmic gymnastics Sports dance 1990, n=64 1997, n=52 Men, n=13	Judo Karate Wrestling 1990, n=41 1997, n=53 Men, n=79	1997, n=10 Men, n=37	Badminton **Hockey** ***Basketball*** Soccer Table tennis Team handball **Tennis** **Volleyball** Underwater r ugby 1990, n=183 1997, n=252 Men, n=277	Discus Javelin Power lifting Shot put Sprints 1990, n=17 1997, n=31 Men, n=18	1990,n=522 1997,n=572 Men, n=687	1990,n=448 1997,n=574 Men, n=629
% ED, Women									
1990	14%	20%	35%	29%	--	12%	0%	18%	5%
1997	17%	24%	42%	30%	10%	16%	3%	20%	9%
Australia		30.9% (n=94)				8.2% (n=61)			5.5% (n=629)
% ED, Men									
1997	4%	9%	0%	18%	22%	5%	<0.5%	8%	0.5%
Australia		6.0% (n=55)				0% (n=53)			0% (n=108)

† Sundgot-Borgen J, Torstveit ML. Prevalence of eating disorders in elite female athletes. *Int J Sport Nutr* 1993; 3:29-40.
‡ Sundgot-Borgen J, Torstveit MK. Prevalence of eating disorders in elite athletes is higher than in the general population. *Clin J Sport Med* 2004; 14: 25-32.
§Byrne S, McLean N. Elite athletes: effects of the pressure to be thin. *J Sci Med Sport* 2002; 16: 230-234.
*Sports considered in the Australian study are bolded; numbers for the Australian study are given in the table.
**Anti-gravitation sports were added to the 1997 Norway study, but a list of the sports that comprise this category was not given.

In a meta-analysis of 34 controlled studies, Smolak, Murnen, and Ruble (2000) found that elite athletes in sports emphasizing thinness were at increased risk of eating problems, as measured by the EDI drive for thinness scale, the EDI body dissatisfaction scale, or a similar measure [35]. However, non-elite athletes, especially in high school, had a reduced risk of eating problems; and runners, gymnasts, and swimmers—typically considered high-risk groups for ED—had similar eating problems to controls. These results may be confounded by the reliance on body dissatisfaction as a measure of ED; body dissatisfaction was lower in athletes in every study where it was reported, but body dissatisfaction may not be a fundamental feature of ED in athletes (see measurement, above). Combining body dissatisfaction with drive for thinness may have masked elevated drive for thinness in the athletes. Still, it appears that, in some cases, sports may actually reduce the risk of ED in young, non-elite women athletes by increasing their self-esteem and body satisfaction.

A study of athletes on national teams in Finland [60] found that the prevalence of female athletes with elevated weight and diet concerns was low: 13% in weight-class athletes versus 11% in controls and 0% in endurance athletes. However, there are several concerns with the study's validity: weight and diet concerns were measured simply as a combination of EDI scores on body dissatisfaction—which was lower in athletes—and drive for thinness—which was higher in athletes; also, participation rates were not given but appear exceedingly low: all athletes in the national training teams were invited to participate (total number was not given), but only 173 women participated; finally scores on the EDI were similar in males and females, an unexpected finding. Also, though no female endurance athletes were classified as at-risk for ED, they had the highest levels of menstrual irregularity in the sample (41%). Given the strong link between disordered eating and menstrual irregularity, this suggests that endurance athletes underreported ED or that the screening tool for ED risk had low sensitivity.

The most informative studies have estimated the prevalence of ED using DSM-IV criteria. A nationwide survey of elite distance runners in Britain [61] found a 16% prevalence of AN (3.9%), BN (1.1%), or EDNOS (11%), which is presumably higher than expected for similarly aged, non-athletic women, but the study lacked an appropriate control group. A survey of 562 female athletes from NCAA division I teams [25] found a 13.15% prevalence of AN (0%), BN (1.1%), or EDNOS (12.05%), but also lacked a control group, making it impossible to tell if these rates are elevated compared with the general population of college women. The study also combined athletes from 9 different sports, a quarter of whom were swimmers, and thus could not estimate prevalence for different sports types. A study of 113 non-elite ballet dancers found a 26.6% prevalence of AN (1.8%), BN (2.7%), or EDNOS (22.1%), which was higher than controls [50].

The best estimates of prevalence of AN, BN, and EDNOS in elite female athletes come from the aforementioned prevalence studies from Norway [11,27] and Australia [37] (Table 1). In the more recent Norwegian study, female athletes had a 2.2-fold increase in risk of ED compared with non-athletes (20% vs. 9%). Risk was elevated in every sport type except power sports. Risk increased in all athlete groups and in controls from 1990 to 1997, indicating that ED are increasing in the general population. Athletes in sports with a weight-class or sports that emphasize leanness (aesthetic, endurance) were at highest risk of ED. The prevalence of AN, BN, or EDNOS in the 1997 control group (9%) was similar to the 8.7%

prevalence found in a large 1995 population-based study of ED in women in Norway [62], adding credence to the study.

In the Australian study, female athletes in thin-build sports had a 5.6-fold increase in risk of ED (30.9% vs. 5.8%), but female athletes in normal-build sports had only a 1.4-fold increase in risk (8.2% vs. 5.8%). The 30.9% prevalence of ED in thin-build sports agrees with the 24-42% prevalence range in the corresponding aesthetic, endurance, and weight-class sports of the Norwegian study. The 8.2% prevalence of ED in normal-build sports appears to contrast the 16% prevalence of ED in the corresponding ball sports category of the Norwegian study; however, the relative risks (relative to controls) are similar for the two studies: 1.4 for normal build sports in the Australian study and 1.8 for ball sports in the Norwegian study. Overall, we can conclude that, compared with non-athletes, elite female athletes in endurance, aesthetic, and weight class sports have a 2.7-5.6-fold increased risk of ED and elite female athletes in ball-game sports have a 1.4-1.8 fold increased risk of ED.

Further evidence of an increased prevalence of ED in female athletes compared with non-athletes may be inferred from studies that have measured menstrual irregularity in athletes. Studies have unequivocally shown a higher rate of menstrual irregularity in female athletes than in the general population, particularly in weight-dependent sports [41,55,60,63-65]. Menstrual irregularity in athletes may be a marker for disordered eating, as energy deficit is the major etiologic factor in the development of athletic amenorrhea. It seems unlikely that the observed excess of menstrual irregularity in athletes can be explained entirely by involuntary energy deficit.

Female Athlete Triad

Few studies have attempted to measure the prevalence of female athlete triad, though many studies have measured ED or menstrual irregularity in athletes. The prevalence of ED is reviewed above. Recent estimates of the prevalence of current menstrual irregularity (oligomenorrhea or amenorrhea) in athletes range from 18%-48%, depending on the level and type of athletes being measured [41,55,60,63-65]. Few studies have attempted to estimate the prevalence of osteopenia or osteoporosis in female athletes. Some studies have tried to use stress fractures as a marker of bone demineralization [55,65], but the results are difficult to interpret because a stress fracture is not necessarily a marker of low bone mass. Klugland, Sundgot-Borgen, and Steffan (2001) estimated a 4.5% prevalence of full-blown female athlete triad (osteopenia/osteoporosis, ED, and menstrual irregularity) in elite athletes in Norway [66]. Athletes in endurance sports were at highest risk. Osteopenia was seen less frequently than the other two components of the triad (6% had osteopenia, 23.5% had ED, and 31.6% had menstrual irregularity). A high proportion of ED in this sample were bulimia or subclinical bulimia, and bulimic behaviors are less likely to result in osteopenia than anorectic behaviors [67]. Thus, prevalence studies of female athlete triad should screen specifically for restrictive eating behaviors and menstrual irregularity. More studies should measure bone density to quantify the risk of female athlete triad.

Male Athletes

Eating disorders are relatively rare in men compared with women and, correspondingly, are less prevalent in male athletes than in female athletes [27,42]. Thus, male athletes have been largely ignored in studies of ED in athletes. The few studies that have been conducted were generally small, considered a single high-risk sport, and lacked an adequate control group. These studies focused largely on the rapid weight loss techniques and frequent weight cycling that occur in sports with a weight class. Athletes trying to "make weight" may use fasting, excessive running, saunas, rubber suits, vomiting, laxatives, and diuretics, to rapidly lose weight. These practices can cause severe dehydration and even death: three NCAA wrestlers died from dehydration and heart failure in 1997 [68]. Prolonged attention to weight and dieting and frequent weight cycling may also lead to the development of ED. Studies that have examined wrestlers [69-76], lightweight rowers [72,77], male jockeys [78-79], swimmers [44], cross country runners [80], lightweight football players [81] have either found higher rates of dangerous rapid weight loss techniques [69,71,75-79], weight cycling [71,75-77], disordered eating behaviors [75-76,81], or weight and eating concerns [70-72,74,78,80-81] compared with either a non-weight dependent sport such as football or an assumed minimal level of these behaviors and attitudes in non-athletic men. As many as three-quarters of jockeys and wrestlers reported the use of at least one potentially harmful weight loss method [76,78-79]. One study reported that 35% of college wrestlers had lost 2-10 pounds more than 100 times [71].

While these studies are worthy of note and suggest an increased risk of eating disturbances in certain male sports, the data are difficult to interpret without appropriate control groups. Certain potentially dangerous eating behaviors may be common in weight-dependent sports, but these behaviors may not extend beyond the competitive season. Unlike women, men face fewer pressures to maintain an abnormally low weight outside of the context of their sport. Dale and Landers (1999) found that disordered attitudes and behaviors regarding food and weight abated after the wrestling season ended [74]. A Finnish study of national caliber male athletes in many sports [60] found athletes reporting weight reduction was high in weight class sports (93%), but the prevalence of subjects with elevated weight and diet concerns based on self-report was low in all sports (0-5%) and was similar to controls, though problems with this study are noted above.

Few studies have estimated the prevalence of AN, BN, and ENDOS in male athletes. A statewide survey of high school wrestlers in Wisconsin [76] found a 1.7% prevalence of BN, which is presumably higher than expected for young men, but the study lacked a comparison group. A study of 883 male athletes from NCAA Division I athletic teams failed to find an elevated rate of AN (0%), BN (0%), or EDNOS (.1%), though 2% admitted purging (vomiting, laxatives, or diuretics) on a weekly basis [25]; 38% were identified as at-risk for BN, and 9.5% as at-risk for AN. However, no control group was used. These results are difficult to interpret because the researchers applied overly strict criteria for AN, BN, and EDNOS—for example, a BMI of less than 15 kg/m^2 was an absolute criteria of the diagnosis of AN—and overly lenient criteria for "at-risk" athletes—for example, a BMI of less than 20 kg/m^2 or infrequent binge eating qualified an athlete as at-risk. The study also grouped data from 10 divergent sports, and football players made up more than one-third of the sample. Wrestlers were identified as being at higher risk than other sports.

The Norwegian [27] and Australian [37] prevalence studies are the only large-scale, controlled studies of ED in male athletes to estimate AN, BN, and EDNOS (Table 1). In the Norwegian study, elite male athletes had a 16-fold higher prevalence of ED than male controls (8% vs. 0.5%). Men in anti-gravitation sports (22%), weight class sports (18%), and endurance (9%) sports were at highest risk for ED, but athletes in ballgame sports also had 10-fold elevated risks compared with controls (5% vs. 0.5%). In the Australian study, 6% of male athletes in thin-build sports had ED, but no controls had ED, making it impossible to calculate a relative risk. Unlike the Norwegian study, the Australian study found no cases of ED in male athletes in normal-build sports (ball game sports). However, the Australian study only sampled 53 men in normal build sports, and even if prevalence of ED were 5%, a sample of 53 would be expected to yield few cases (in fact, there would be a 7% chance of detecting no cases). Thus, the Australian study had insufficient power to detect a difference between male athletes in normal-build sports and controls.

Interestingly, in both studies, men in weight-dependent sports have similar rates of ED as female controls. In the Norwegian study, male athletes in all sports combined have a 16-fold increased risk of ED relative to non-athletes, but female athletes have only a 2.2-fold relative risk. Weight-dependent sports may represent one of the few pressures that compel men to maintain an abnormally low weight (in contrast to the countless socio-cultural pressures that compel women). If so, participation in weight-dependent sports may account for a considerable proportion of the eating disorders seen in men. For example, in a study of male and female patients with AN and BN, 37% of the men had been involved in a sport or occupation in which weight was essential for good performance, compared with only 13% of the women [82].

In summary, elite male athletes appear to be at a significantly increased risk of ED compared with men in the general population, particularly elite athletes in anti-gravitation, weight class, or endurance sports. Participation in weight-dependent sports could be the cause of a large proportion of the ED seen in men. More studies using the two-stage method of Sundgot-Borgen and Torstveit (2004) are needed to help establish the prevalence of ED in both elite and non-elite male athletes.

Risk Factors

Risk factors for ED in athletes may be intrinsic to the sport (sport-dependent) or to the athlete (sport-independent). Sports expose athletes to unique risk factors for ED, such as pressure from coaches, drive to win, and weight cycling. Alternatively, individuals with an existent or emerging eating disorder may be attracted to sports to lose weight, justify their emerging eating patterns, or hide their eating disorder; and individuals with personality traits that help them excel in athletics—e.g., high-achieving, perfectionist, disciplined—may be at higher risk of ED independent of sport. The development of ED is likely multi-factorial, involving both sport-dependent and sport-independent factors; for example, a coach's reprimand could initiate an eating disorder in a gymnast who was already weight conscious and driven to succeed.

Most risk factor studies are cross-sectional and many mistake co-morbidities and outcomes for causes. For example, studies have reported higher substance abuse, depression, and suicide attempts [83] and higher rates of detachment, anxiety, and hostility [84] in athletes with ED, but these behaviors may be results, rather than causes, of ED. Longitudinal studies are needed to definitively establish risk factors for ED in athletes.

Sport-Dependent Factors

The Culture of Sport

Athletes who believe that thinness confers an advantage in their sport are highly motivated to diet. In a study by Sundgot-Borgen (1994), 100% of dieting athletes with ED said they were dieting to improve performance, but only 40% said they were dieting to improve appearance [85]. If initial weight loss is rewarded with gains in performance, this may reinforce the athlete's perception that weight loss is beneficial and may precipitate an eating disorder.

Coaches may strongly influence an athlete’s outlook, self-esteem, and choices. Sundgot-Borgen found that 30% of elite athletes with ED identified the loss or change of a coach as an initiating factor of their ED [85]. Coaches who believe that thinness confers an advantage may pressure athletes to lose weight. Sundgot-Borgen found that 67% of dieting athletes with ED had begun dieting at the recommendation of their coach [85].

The behaviors and appearance of teammates and competitors may also promote unhealthy eating patterns. If several athletes take drastic measures to lose weight or are obviously emaciated, a culture develops that perpetuates the problem. As with performance-enhancing drugs, if it seems that "everyone is doing it," then athletes may believe that being abnormally thin is expected and necessary for success.

Chronic Dieting, Weight Loss, and Weight Cycling

Several lines of evidence suggest that dieting plays a strong role in the development of ED. Prospective studies have linked dieting to the development of eating disorders in non-athletes [86-88]. Hsu (1990) proposed that the prevalence of ED is directly proportional to the prevalence of dieting behavior in a given community, which is consistent with the high prevalence of ED in athletes in weight-dependent sports, who are under pressure to diet for performance or to make weight [89]. The exact relationship between dieting and ED is unknown, but dieting may cause both psychological and biochemical changes that precipitate ED. Prolonged periods of calorie restriction or weight fluctuations may cause multiple endocrine and metabolic changes that interfere with mood and the ability to recognize satiation or hunger (food regulation).

Unsupervised weight loss, in particular, may be a risk factor for ED [85]. Athletes who are forced to rest because of injury or illness may fear weight gain and feel that they must greatly restrict their calories. This period of calorie restriction may also precipitate an ED [85,90].

Physical Activity

Some researchers have hypothesized that exercise plays a central role in the development of AN [90-92]. Epling and Pierce (1996) found that laboratory rats placed on food restriction exercise excessively, decrease their food intake, and starve to death when given access to a running wheel [91]. In contrast, rats placed on food restriction but not given a running wheel adapt to famine conditions by reducing their activity, and they survive. Epling and Pierce suggested that semi-starvation causes hyperactivity, which in turn gives positive biochemical feedback (such as increased endorphin levels), which in turn suppresses the appetite and reduces food intake, thus creating a self-perpetuating cycle of exercise, starvation, and weight loss—termed "activity-induced anorexia." Some evidence suggests that a similar phenomenon may occur in humans. For example, Davis et al. (1994) found that 60% of their sample of 45 ED patients (most of whom had AN) had been competitive athletes prior to the start of dieting [90]. The fact that sport and exercise pre-dated onset of AN may suggest a role of physical activity in the development of ED. Though it is unlikely that physical activity is the sole cause of ED, it may be an important mediator in athletes. Excessive exercise combined with dieting and weight loss may result in physiological and psychological changes that set the stage for the development of ED.

Sport-Independent Factors

Self-Selection

Certain sports may attract athletes with pre-existing ED [93]. A young person who is on the verge of developing an eating disorder may join a sport to lose weight or to justify their behaviors [84]. In this case, then higher rates of ED in athletes may simply reflect self-selection. Researchers have found high rates of ED in fitness instructors, who may have chosen their profession because of preoccupation with weight and shape [94-95]. However, O'Connor et al. (1996) found that weight pre-occupation in college gymnasts increased after they started gymnastics and abated after they ended competition—suggesting that weight pre-occupation was sports-dependent [96]. Overall, though some individuals with ED may join sports, it is unlikely that all eating disordered individuals find themselves playing competitive sports.

Personality Factors

In an interesting, but highly controversial article, Yates, Leehey, and Shisslak (1983) compared "obligatory" male runners—a group of middle-aged marathoners and trail runners who had purportedly tied their identities to obsessive, habitual running—to anorectic teenage women, noting similarities in personality traits, conflicts, adaptive styles, and behaviors [97]:

> Anorexic women and members of their families are often compulsively athletic, and obligatory runners may demonstrate a bizarre preoccupation with food and an unusual emphasis on lean body mass. We speculate that both phenomena could represent a partially successful—albeit dangerous—attempt to establish an identity. p.251

Yates, Leehey, and Shisslak speculated that long distance running and eating disorders are two manifestations of a common psychopathology. Though they may have overstated the pathology of the obligatory runners, their observation of common personality factors in ED patients and athletes is on the mark. Certain personality factors that are common in athletes—that may indeed be instrumental in their athletic success—may predispose them to ED. Athletes are often competitive, achievement-oriented, disciplined, obsessive, and perfectionistic, characteristics commonly seen in individuals with ED. Both athletes and individuals with ED may also have low self-esteem and an underdeveloped or overly narrow sense of identity [25,98]. Longitudinal studies are needed to see if such personality factors in athletes predict who will get ED. Certain personality factors likely interact with sport-specific triggers to lead to ED in athletes. Existing psychopathologic conditions such as obsessive-compulsive disorder may also lead to ED [99], but these conditions may not be more common in athletes than non-athletes.

Body Type

Some researchers have proposed that the larger the disparity between an athlete's body type and his/her sport's perceived ideal body type, the higher the risk of ED. Athletes may pick the wrong sport for their adult body type if they specialize before puberty [85]. Hamilton et al. (1988) found that ballerinas from less selective dance companies had more eating problems and a greater familial history of obesity than ballerinas from more selective dance companies, though both groups averaged 14% below their ideal weight [100]. The authors suggest that dancers who have survived a stringent process of early selection may be more naturally suited to the body type demanded by ballet and are thus at less risk for ED. Though logical, this would imply that the most successful athletes would be at lowest risk of ED, an empirical finding that has not manifest in the literature.

Risk Factors for the Female Athlete Triad

Since an eating disorder (or involuntary energy deficit) is the initiating factor of the female athlete triad, the risk factors for female athlete triad are similar to those for ED in athletes. However, restrictive disordered eating is more likely than binge/purge behaviors to cause menstrual irregularity and bone loss, so risk factors for the female athlete triad are specifically those risk factors that lead to anorectic behaviors. Though studies of athletes have not distinguished between risk factors for AN and risk factors for BN, in non-athletes, obsessive-compulsive disorder and perfectionism appear to be specific risk factors for AN and childhood or parental obesity and social phobia appear to be specific risk factors for BN [99]. It is unclear if these distinctions extend to athletes. Sports that stress a high degree of lean mass (power and strength sports) or involve high-impact movements may also protect against bone loss even if a restrictive ED is present. For example, studies of gymnasts show that high-impact, bone-stimulating exercises may override the negative effects of disordered eating and menstrual irregularity on the skeleton [101-102]. The female athlete triad may be more common in sports with repetitive, low-impact loading on the skeleton, such as running.

Outcomes

The short-term (acute) and long-term consequences of ED in athletes have not been well studied [103]. The majority of studies have focused on the female athlete triad and either skeletal deficits or fractures; even these studies have followed athletes for a limited amount of time. More studies are needed to characterize the long-term health consequences of sub-clinical and clinical ED in athletes, including physiologic and skeletal effects, psychological effects, mortality, and effects on general well being.

In moving from the epidemiologic to the clinical literature, it will be useful to describe another case report that illustrates the potential severity and intractability of ED in athletes.

Case Report 2

Warren et al. (1990) report a case of femoral head collapse and short stature in a 20-year old ballerina. The woman had begun to dance at 8 years of age and developed full-blown AN at 11 years [104]. After treatment, she regained weight to 54.5 kg by age 13, but then continued to battle AN, including three hospitalizations. At age 20, she weighed 34 kg and was only 1.5 meters tall (BMI: 15.1 kg/m^2), less than her expected height. X-rays revealed femoral head collapse and severe osteoporosis. Nutritional counseling and estrogen replacement were recommended but the patient refused medical treatment. The patient needed a hip replacement, but, at last report, her nutritional status was insufficient to permit surgery.

Skeletal Effects in Women

For women, the majority of bone accrual occurs between the ages of 11 and 14 years, and 90% of peak bone mass is achieved by age 16 [105]. Malnutrition and hypoestrogenism that interrupt this critical window may significantly halt skeletal growth. Pre- and peripubertal girls with delayed menarche (primary amenorrhea) may fail to properly accrue bone mass, and postpubertal girls with secondary amenorrhea or oligomenorrhea may lose bone mass. Women with primary amenorrhea have larger deficits in bone mass and density than women with secondary amenorrhea [106]. At the extreme, some women athletes and anorectics in their twenties and thirties have bone densities that would be comparable to a 70- or 80-year-old woman [8,104]. Earlier age of onset of AN is associated with deficits in bone size, which also predispose to increased fragility [107].

Women who recover from ED gain bone, but fail to recover bone mass and density to normal levels. There may be a catch-up effect whereby women who recover from ED may be able to accumulate bone during their late teens or even during their twenties [108-109]. A few studies show normal levels of bone density in former elite athletes [110] and former anorectics [111] 25 years after retirement and 11 years after initial diagnosis, respectively; however, these studies are cross-sectional, and we cannot conclude that these women regained bone after initial deficits. Longitudinal studies in athletes show that bone deficits due to amenorrhea are largely irreversible [112-115]. Women in their early twenties who spontaneously regained menses improved lumbar spine bone density by 12%-17%, but still remained critically below normal [112-114]. Eight years after resumption of menses, formerly amenorrheic ballet dancers still had spine bone density 15% below controls [115]. Longitudinal studies of bone density in anorectics are confounded by the chronic nature of the disease, but also show severe bone deficits after recovery [116-118]; estimates of bone deficits at the spine and hip range from 7%-31% (mean 15%) [118].

The best evidence of sustained deficits in bone density and quality come from long-term studies of fracture risk. Women with a history of AN show a 2-3-fold increase in overall incidence of fracture, and up to a 5-fold increase in incidence of vertebral and hip fracture as many as 60 years past diagnosis [117-120]. Bone deficits may be less drastic in women with a history of EDNOS, but researchers estimate a 2-fold increase in incidence of fracture, with higher risks at the spine and hip [117-118]. EDNOS is a heterogeneous category, and certain subgroups, such as women with subclinical AN, may have even higher risks. Women with female athlete triad who have weight reductions and duration of amenorrhea similar to anorectic women are likely to have reductions in BMD and fracture risk similar to women with AN [8,104], but exercise may offer some protection against bone loss or may be associated with favorable geometric changes that increase bone strength [121]. Long-term fracture risk in formerly amenorrheic athletes is unknown, and it will be several more decades before this can be evaluated, since the female athlete triad is a recently recognized syndrome [6]. We do know that gymnasts are protected against long-term bone loss and osteoporotic fractures because of their high-impact exercise [101-102]. It is unclear if adolescent gymnasts stunt their vertebral growth [122-123].

Skeletal Effects in Men

Men have a larger window of skeletal growth, and continue to gain significant bone mass until 20 years of age [105]; thus men who suffer from AN in adolescence might have a larger window of opportunity than women to catch up to peak bone mass. However, men in the acute stages of AN have similar levels of osteoporosis and fracture as their female counterparts [124-126]. Estimates of relative fracture incidence in men with a history of AN are similar to those of women, but are based on small sample sizes. It is unknown whether male athletes suffer from a syndrome similar to the female athlete triad, with reduced testosterone levels and osteopenia, but a few studies have seen moderate reductions in lumbar spine BMD in male distance runners with high training volumes [127-128].

Injuries/Detriments to Performance

Women athletes with amenorrhea may have higher rates of stress fractures and scoliosis [129-131], likely secondary to reduced bone density and accelerated bone resorption. Rapid weight loss in wrestlers causes dehydration and acutely decreases upper body strength, power, and anaerobic and aerobic capacity [132-134], though these effects appear transitory.

Weight cycling in wrestlers may reduce metabolic rate and increase body fat, though the longevity of these effects are unclear [135]. Eating disorders result in energy deficits, electrolyte imbalance, fatigue, and muscle wasting—all of which could clearly hurt performance; however, athletes with ED are often able to perform at an extraordinarily high level for their nutritional status, adding to the denial surrounding ED in athletes.

Mortality

AN and BN have high mortality rates for psychiatric disorders [136]. Rapid weight loss can also cause sudden death in athletes. In 1997, three NCAA male wrestlers died of hyperthermia and cardiorespiratory arrest while trying to make weight [68].

Residual Psychological Effects/Co-Morbidities

Recovery from ED is often difficult and prolonged. Ratnasuriya et al. (1991) found continued anorectic behavior, continued difficulties with weight and food, and poor social adjustment in a cohort of formerly anorexic patients 20 years after diagnosis [137]. Iacovino (2004) found higher rates of depression and alcoholism in former anorectics [138]. The course of illness and recovery in athletes with ED has not been well documented. Holderness, Brooks-Gunn, and Warren (1994) found high levels of emotional stress and substance abuse in non-athletes with ED, but not in ballet students with ED [139]. In contrast, cases of depression and hysteria have been documented in ballet dancers with ED [140]. Gutgesell and Timmerman found increased alcohol abuse in runners with a history of BN [141]. Longitudinal studies are needed before we can make conclusions about the long-term psychological effects of ED in athletes. At this point, it seems clear that ED can cause severe emotional stress, at least acutely.

Screening and Prevention

Most research on screening and prevention of ED in athletes has focused on women, so this section will focus on women. Few controlled studies have formally evaluated prevention programs for women, so this section will also propose novel prevention strategies based on the epidemiologic literature on risk factors and outcomes.

Women are at the highest risk for developing ED during adolescence [142-143], and ED symptoms and attitudes appear to be firmly established before college [143]. Since adolescence also is the critical window for achieving peak bone mass [105], educational and psychosocial efforts to prevent ED in female athletes should focus on age group, middle school, and high school athletes. To date, however, research on ED in athletes has focused on screening and intervention programs in college-aged athletes or older [14,65,114,144], when it may be too late for the skeleton. More research is needed on prevention and screening programs for younger athletes.

Screening

Early intervention is critical to preventing negative health outcomes in athletes with ED. All athletes participating in collegiate and interscholastic sports should be screened for ED. Currently, screening for ED is inadequate at the college level [144-145]; screening has not been well studied at the high school level, but is likely inadequate as well.

Detecting ED in an athlete is difficult because of the secretive nature of the disease [28]. Vaughan, King, Cottrell (2004) found that though 91% of collegiate athletic trainers surveyed had dealt with a female athlete with ED, only 27% felt confident in identifying a female athlete with ED [145]. The pre-participation exam is the best chance for widespread screening of athletes. However, there are no evidence-based screening procedures that reliably identify ED in athletes [146], and athletes may be reluctant to answer questions about ED during this exam [147].

Team physicians and trainers should have a high index of suspicion for ED in female athletes, particularly if a woman presents with a stress fracture or menstrual irregularity [28]. Other signs of ED include emaciation, lanugo, bradycardia, and thinning hair (AN) and tooth erosion, edema, gastrointestinal complaints, bloodshot eyes, and swollen parotid glands (BN).

Education

Prevention education should focus on educating athletes and coaches on proper nutrition and on the consequences of ED. Many young women are unaware of the potential harms of ED and amenorrhea, particularly harms to their skeletons. In one survey of college athletes, 70% of the women who were engaging in pathogenic weight-control behaviors thought these behaviors were harmless [43]. A more recent study in Brazil found that 27% of coaches still recommend deleterious weight control practices [148]. Awareness of the severe long-term consequences of ED might prevent coaches from advocating and athletes from initiating these behaviors.

Education should also try to change the message that "thinness=athletic success" to a message that healthy eating and sufficient calories yield strength and endurance, whereas dieting and purging make the body weak and ineffective. Restrictive eating and abnormal eating patterns may also increase body fat relative to muscle mass [149].

Supervised Weight Loss

Unsupervised weight loss may be a risk factor for ED [85]. If an athlete needs to lose weight, a trainer, nutritionist, or physician should provide a weight loss plan and should carefully monitor progress; they should watch for weight loss that is too rapid (more than 1-2 pounds per week) and weight loss that continues after goal weight has been achieved. Coaches should also be sensitive to the effect that dieting athletes may have on team members, particularly on college teams, where athletes often eat together. If a coach openly recommends weight loss for some members of the team, other athletes may perceive a need to lose weight, and may initiate a weight-loss program without supervision.

Changing the Rules

Sports governing bodies can remove incentives that encourage ED by changing the rules of sport. For example, following the death of 3 male collegiate wrestlers in 1997, the NCAA began prohibiting rapid weight loss techniques and moved the time of weigh-in closer to the time of competition. These new policies appear to have been successful in changing college wrestlers' weight loss practices [73].

Preventing Female Athlete Triad

Research should also focus on interventions that prevent bone loss when menstrual irregularity and disordered eating are present, since it is unrealistic to expect that these risk factors will disappear from women's athletics. Mechanical loading is an important determinant of bone mass, architecture, and structural strength [150-156]. Studies of gymnasts show that high-impact, bone-stimulating exercises may override the negative effects to bone that come from disordered eating and menstrual irregularity [101-102]. Thus, it is possible that a properly designed osteogenic exercise program could mitigate bone loss in female athletes who have the other 2 disorders of the female athlete triad.

Previous studies have reported that athletes engaged in sports that produce high strain rates via versatile impact-type movements (eg, soccer) have higher bone mass (9%-40%), better geometry and stronger structure (the largest differences more than 50%) than do either sedentary controls or athletes engaged in sports with lower strain rates and limited movements (eg, running) [155]. Adaptation to this loading seems to occur in a site-specific fashion by gross-geometric changes, structural or architectural changes or by their combination. Clinical trials [151-152] and animal studies [150] also support the high-impact loading concept. Consequently, the important components of osteogenic exercise stimulus are high strain rates (speed and power) and high peak forces in versatile movements. Since the immature skeleton has greater capacity to deposit new bone than mature bone [121,152,156], introduction of these exercises at an early age (ie, prior to college) is critical for optimal benefits.

Treatment

Recommendations for treating ED in athletes are often based on an individual physician's clinical expertise, experience, and judgment, rather than on evidence from clinical studies [93, 157], reflecting the lack of research in this area and the need for flexibility in treating ED. Treatment of athletes with ED may be a team effort, involving a physician, nutritionist, psychiatrist or counselor, and coach [93]. Athletes with ED should be encouraged to increase caloric intake and/or reduce training until menses resume, to intake adequate calcium and vitamin D, and to engage in osteogenic, weight-bearing exercise where appropriate (see prevention above). They should also be given counseling as necessary to treat the psychological aspects of the disease, and some may respond to treatment with anti-depressants. Athletes may need to be withheld from competition and/or participation if they refuse to comply with treatment or if their symptoms are severe enough. The literature on treatments for ED in athletes is sparse, and most controlled studies of ED in athletes have focused on pharmacologic treatments for osteoporosis and osteopenia in female athlete triad and AN.

Pharmacologic Treatments for Osteopenia/Osteoporosis in ED

The optimal treatment for osteopenia/osteoporosis in ED is weight gain and resumption of menses. However, ED is often chronic and treatment can be prolonged. There is a need for pharmacologic agents that can attenuate bone loss or increase bone density in women with active ED and female athlete triad. For better or worse, physicians have conventionally treated amenorrheic athletes with hormone replacement, either post-menopausal hormone therapies such as Premarin plus Provera or oral contraceptives. If bone loss in ED is due to an estrogen deficit, it seems logical that estrogen replacement could reverse this deficit, but the empirical data are unpersuasive. Nutritional deficiencies may play a larger role in bone loss than sex steroids. Hormone replacement—which suppresses bone resorption—may be insufficient for preserving bone mass in women with ED, who have both increased bone resorption and decreased bone formation (unlike post-menopausal women, who predominantly face accelerated bone resorption) [12].

The authors of three longitudinal studies of bone density and estrogen-supplementation in amenorrheic athletes concluded that estrogen supplementation may be warranted [158-160]. However, Braam et al. (2003) failed to include a group of amenorrheic athletes taking oral contraceptives [158], and Rickenlund et al. (2000) failed to include a control group of amenorrheic athletes not taking oral contraceptives [159]; in both cases, observed changes in BMD in oral contraceptive users were small, suggesting little clinically meaningful effect. The most promising study showed an 8% increase in spine BMD in 8 amenorrheic runners with osteopenia who took hormone replacement therapy for 24-30 months compared with a slight loss in spine BMD in 5 amenorrheic runners who refused medication during the same time period [160]. Unfortunately, it is unclear if the observed gains were due to hormone replacement therapy or to other factors; the women who opted for treatment may have been motivated to reverse their osteopenia, and may have also changed their diet and gained weight. This information was not given. At least, we can conclude that estrogen supplementation did not prevent bone gain. Longitudinal studies in non-athletes with AN have also shown only minor effect for oral contraceptives [161-162], even at higher doses of estrogen and for younger ages.

There have only been two randomized clinical trials of oral contraceptives in amenorrheic athletes. Warren et al. (2003) conducted a 2-year placebo-controlled trial of hormone replacement therapy in 24 amenorrheic dancers, and saw no difference in changes in bone density between treatment and placebo [114]. Gibson et al. (1999) conducted a pilot randomized trial of hormone replacement in 34 elite middle and distance runners [163]. There was a relative 1.5% increase in spine BMD in runners on HRT compared with controls. However, the ability to see differences between the two groups was partly obscured by non-compliance in the treatment group and spontaneous resumption of menses in the control group. Two randomized trials in patients with AN showed no effects for HRT or oral contraceptives, respectively [164-165].

Overall, oral contraceptives and hormone replacement therapy appear to confer minimal gains in bone density compared with no treatment. In the absence of weight gain, hormone replacement is unlikely to protect against continued bone loss or to reverse bone deficits. In fact, it may be prudent to recommend against the use of hormone replacement because women may falsely believe that their bones are being protected and may delay weight gain [166-167]. Additionally, the spontaneous return of menses is a good benchmark of improved nutrition.

We cannot rule out that different dosages or different routes of administration of hormone replacement might have more beneficial effects on the skeleton. For example, isolated case reports suggest transdermal estrogen may confer more benefits to bone than oral estrogen, at least some patients [8, 168]. Hormone replacement might also acutely protect against fractures by decreasing bone resorption, even if it does not yield a significant increase in bone density, but data on the effect of estrogen replacement on fractures or stress fractures in this population are not yet available.

Interestingly, doctors have overwhelmingly prescribed estrogen replacement in cases of athletic amenorrhea or ED in the past decade, despite lack of hard evidence of its efficacy. For example, in a 1995 survey, 92% of sports medicine doctors and family physicians reported prescribing estrogen replacement to treat athletic amenorrhea. [169]; in a 2000 survey of pediatricians, sports medicine doctors, and general practitioners, 77.6% reported prescribing hormone replacement therapy to reduce the risk of osteopenia in teenage girls with AN [166]. It is unclear if prescribing practices have changed in light of the handful of studies that have been published in the last decade that show a relative lack of efficacy of hormone replacement therapy in preserving bone when nutritional deficits exist. Interestingly, recent medical school graduates were less likely to report prescribing hormone replacement in AN in the 2000 survey, possibly reflecting changing prescribing practices and greater attention to evidence-based medicine.

Other experimental pharmacologic agents that have been used to treat osteopenia/osteoporosis in ED include DHEA [170], IGF-I [165], recombinant leptin [171], and bisphosphonates [172]. In a non-randomized trial of leptin, 8 women with amenorrhea experienced increases in bone formation markers; several resumed menses, and three had ovulatory cycles. Bone density changes were not measured. In a randomized trial of bisphosphonates, patients who received risedronate had spine bone density increases of 4.1% in 6 months and 4.9% in 9 months in, whereas controls lost bone. This is the first study to show marked increases in bone density in patients with AN without weight gain. However, the women in this study were in their mid-to-late twenties. Bisphosphonates work by decreasing bone resorption rather than enhancing bone formation; therefore may not be helpful in adolescent patients who need to form bone. Also, the long-term risks of bisphosphonates have not been studied in this age group. Bisphosphonates have a long half-life and their effect on future reproductive events and long-term bone quality are unknown, and some reports have questioned their used in children [173]. Further randomized trials are needed to test these promising leads.

Conclusion

Elite male and female athletes in endurance, aesthetic, and weight class sports are at higher risk of ED than the general population. Participation in weight-dependent sports may represent a major risk factor for ED in men. Future prevalence studies should use a two-stage design that sends men and women with high weight and food concerns and women with menstrual irregularity (determined by self-report) to a second-stage structured clinical interview. These studies should specifically aim to identify cases of AN, BN, EDNOS, or female athlete triad and should include a non-athletic control group. Studies that measure bone density are needed to estimate the prevalence of female athlete triad in specific athletic populations. Longitudinal studies are needed to determine specific risk factors for ED in athletes.

Skeletal effects dominate the research on outcomes of ED in athletes. Male and female athletes with ED are at risk for severe bone deficits and early osteoporosis. Athletes with ED may resist identification and treatment; and recovery from ED can be prolonged. Early intervention is critical to preventing negative health outcomes. Prevention strategies should target athletes before college, since ED may begin before college and critical skeletal development occurs during early adolescence. High-impact exercise during adolescence has the potential to mitigate bone loss due to ED, but studies are needed to test this hypothesis. Evidence does not support the use of hormone replacement therapy to restore bone mass in athletes with ED and osteopenia. Priorities for research on ED in athletes include research on prevention and screening strategies in adolescent and college athletes and treatments for osteopenia and osteoporosis in athletes with established ED and female athlete triad.

References

[1] Garner DM, Garfinkel PE. Socio-cultural factors in the development of anorexia nervosa. *Psychol. Med.* 1980: 10: 647-656.

[2] Maloney MJ. Anorexia and bulimia in dancers.Accurate diagnosis and treatment planning. *Clin. Sports Med.* 1983; 2:549-555.

[3] Szmukler GI, Eisler I, Gillies C, Hayward ME. The implications of anorexia nervosa in a ballet school. *J. Psychiatr. Res.* 1985; 19:177-181.

[4] Braisted JR, Mellin L, Gong EJ, Irwin CE. The adolescent ballet dancer. Nutritional practices and characteristics associated with anorexia nervosa. *J. Adolesc. Health Care* 1985; 6:365-371.

[5] American Psychiatric Association: Diagnostic and Statistical Manual of Mental Disorders, 3rd edition (DSM-III). Washington, D.C., APA Press, 1980.

[6] Yeager KK, Agostini R, Nattiv A, Drinkwater B. The female athlete triad: disordered eating, amenorrhea, osteoporosis. *Med. Sci. Sports Exerc.* 25:775-777; 1993.

[7] Otis CL, Drinkwater B, Johnson M, Loucks A, Wilmore J. American College of Sports Medicine position stand. the female athlete triad. *Med. Sci. Sports Exerc.* 1997;29:i-ix.

[8] Zanker CL, Cooke CB, Truscott JG, Oldroyd B, Jacobs HS. Annual changes of bone density over 12 years in an amenorrheic athlete. *Med. Sci. Sports Exerc.* 2004;36:137-142.

[9] Johnson MD. Disordered eating in active and athletic women. *Clin. Sports Med.* 1994; 13: 355-369.

[10] American Psychiatric Association: Diagnostic and Statistical Manual of Mental Disorders, 4th edition (DSM-III). Washington, D.C., APA Press, 1994.

[11] Sundgot-Borgen J. Prevalence of eating disorders in elite female athletes. *Int. J. Sport Nutr.* 1993; 3:29-40.

[12] Loucks AB. Introduction to menstrual disturbances in athletes. *Med. Sci. Sports Exerc.* 2003; 35: 1551-1552.

[13] Wilmore JH. Eating and weight disorders in the female athlete. *Int. J. Sport. Nutr.* 1991; 1:104-117.

[14] Cobb KL, Bachrach, LK, Greendale G, Marcus R, Neer R, Nieves J, Sowers MF, Brown BW, Gopalakrishnan G, Luetters C, Tanner HK, Ward B, Kelsey JL. Disordered eating, menstrual irregularity, and bone mineral density in female distance runners. *Med. Sci. Sports Exerc.* 2003; 35:711-719.

[15] Zanker CL, Cooke CB. Energy balance, bone turnover, and skeletal health in physically active individuals. *Med. Sci. Sports Exerc.* 2004; 36:1372-1381.

[16] Williams NI, Helmreich DL, Parfitt DB, Caston-Balderrama A, Cameron JL. Evidence for a causal role of low energy availability in the induction of menstrual cycle disturbances during strenuous exercise training. *J. Clin. Endocrinol. Metab.* 2001; 86:5184-5193.

[17] Warren MP, Voussoughian F, Geer EB, Hyle EP, Adberg CL, Ramos RH. Functional hypothalamic amenorrhea: hypoleptinemia and disordered eating. *J. Clin. Endocrinol. Metab.* 1999; 84:873-877.

[18] De Souza MJ, Williams NI. Physiological aspects of clinical sequelae of energy deficiency and hypoestrogenism in exercising women. *Hum Reprod Update* 2004; 10:433-448.

[19] Loucks AB. Energy availability, not body fatness, regulates reproductive function in women. *Exerc Sport Sci Rev* 2003; 31:144-148.

[20] De Souza MJ, Van Heest J, Demers LM, Lasley BL. Luteal phase deficiency in recreational runners: evidence for a hypometabolic state. *J. Clinic. Endocrinol. Metab.* 2003; 88:337-346.

[21] Garner DM, Garfinkel PE. The eating attitudes test: an index of the symptoms of anorexia nervosa. *Psychol. Med.* 1979; 9: 273-279.

[22] Garner DM, Olmsted MP, BohrY, Garfinkel PE. The eating attitudes test: psychometric features and clinical correlates. *Psychol. Med.* 1982; 12:871-878.

[23] Garner DM, Olmsted MP, Polivy J. Development and validation of a multidimensional eating disorder inventory for anorexia nervosa and bulimia. *Int. J. Eating Disorders* 1983; 2: 15-34.

[24] Garner DM, Olmsted MP. *Manual for eating disorders inventory.* Odessa FL: Psychological Assessment Resources, Inc. 1984.

[25] Johnson C, Powers PS, Dick R. Athletes and eating disorders: the National Collegiate Athletic Association study. *Int. J. Eat. Disord.* 1999; 26: 179-188.

[26] Fairburn CG, Beglin SJ. Assessment of eating disorders: Interview or self-report questionnaire? *Int. J. Eat. Disord.* 1994; 16:363-370.

[27] Sundgot-Borgen J, Torstveit MK. Prevalence of eating disorders in elite athletes is higher than in the general population. *Clin. J. Sport. Med.* 2004; 14:25-32.

[28] Joy E, Clark N, Ireland ML, Martire J, Nattiv A, Varechok S. Team management of the female athlete triad: Part 1: What to look for, what to ask. *Physician. Sportsmed.* 1997; 25.

[29] Stice E, Telch CF, Rizvi SL. Development and validation of the eating disorder diagnostic scale: a brief self-report measure of anorexia, bulimia, and binge-eating disorder. *Psychol. Assess.* 2000; 12:123-131.

[30] Nevonen L, Broberg AG. Validating the Eating Disorder Inventory-2 (EDI-2) in Sweden. *Eat Weight Disord.*2001; 6:59-67.

[31] O'Connor PJ, Lewis RD, Kirchner EM. Eating disorder symptoms in female college gymnasts. *Med. Sci. Sports Exerc.* 1995; 27:550-555.

[32] Black DR, Larkin LJ, Coster DC, Leverenz LJ, Abood DA. Physiologic screening test for eating disorders/disordered eating among female collegiate athletes. *J. Athl. Train.* 2003; 38:286-297.

[33] Golden NH. A review of the female athlete triad (amenorrhea, osteoporosis and disordered eating). *Int J Adolesc Med Health* 2002; 14:9-17.

[34] Walsh JM, Wheat ME, Freund K. Detection, evaluation, and treatment of eating disorders: The role of the primary care physician. *J Gen Intern Med* 2000; 15:557-590.

[35] Smolak L, Murnen SK, Ruble AE. Female athletes and eating problems: a meta-analysis. *Int J Eat Disord* 2000; 27: 371-380.

[36] Beals KA, Manore MM. The prevalence and consequences of subclinical eating disorders in female athletes. *Int. J. Sport. Nutr.* 1994; 4: 175-195.

[37] Byrne S, McLean N. Elite athletes: effects of the pressure to be thin. *J. Sci. Med. Sport.* 2002; 16: 230-234.

[38] Ziegler PJ, Khoo CS, Sherr B, Nelson JA, Larson WM, Drewnoski A. Body image and dieting behaviors among elite figure skaters. *Int. J. Eat. Disord.* 1998; 24:421-427.

[39] Yates A, Edman JD, Crago M, Crowell D. Eating disorder symptoms in runners, cyclists, and paddlers. *Addict. Behav.* 2003; 28:1473-1480.

[40] McNulty KY, Adams CH, Anderson JM, Affenito SG. Development and validation of a screening tool to identify eating disorders in female athletes. *J. Am. Diet. Assoc.* 2001; 101: 886-892.

[41] Hopkinson RA, Lock J. Athletics, perfectionism, and disordered eating. *Eat Weight Disord* 2004; 9:99-106.

[42] Byrne S, McLean N. Eating disorders in athletes: a review of the literature. *J Sci Med Sport* 2001; 4:145-159.

[43] Rosen LW, McKeag DB, Hough DO, Curley V. Pathogenic weight-control behavior in female athletes. *Physician Sportsmed* 1986; 14:79-86.

[44] Dummer GM, Rosen LW, Heusner WW, Roberts PJ, and Counsilman JE. Pathogenic weight-control behaviors of young competitive swimmers. *Physician Sportsmed.* 1987; 15: 75-84.

[45] Rosen LW, Hough DO. Pathogenic weight-control behaviors of female college gymnasts. *Physician Sportsmed.* 1988; 16:140-146.

[46] Evers CL. Dietary intake and symptoms of anorexia nervosa in female university dancers. *J. Am. Diet. Assoc.* 1987; 87:66-68.

[47] Kurtzman FD, Yager J, Landsverk J, Wiesmeier E, Bodurka DC. Eating disorders among selected female student populations at UCLA. *J. Am. Diet. Assoc.* 1989; 89:45-53.

[48] Abraham S. Eating and weight controlling behaviors of young ballet dancers. *Psychopathology* 1996; 29:218-222.

[49] Abraham S. Characteristics of eating disorders among young ballet dancers. *Psychopathology* 1996; 29:223-229.

[50] Ravaldi C, Vannacci A, Zucchi T, Mannucci E, Cabras PL, Boldrini M, Murciano L, Rotella CM, Ricca V. Eating disorders and body image disturbances among ballet dancers, gymnasium users, and body builders. *Psychopathology* 2003; 36: 247-254.

[51] Estok PJ, Rudy EB. The relationship between eating disorders and running in women. *Res. Nurs. Health* 1996; 19: 377-387.

[52] Benson JE, Allemann Y, Theintz GE, Howald H. Eating problems and calorie intake levels in Swiss adolescent athletes. *Int. J. Sports Med.* 1990; 11: 249-252.

[53] Karlson KA, Becker CB, Merkur A. Prevalence of eating disordered behavior in collegiate lightweight women rowers and distance runners. *Clin. J. Sport. Med.* 2001; 11:32-37.

[54] Terry PC, Waite J. Eating attitudes and body shape perceptions among elite rowers: effects of age, gender, and weight category. *Aust. J. Sci. Med. Sport* .1996; 28:3-6.

[55] Beals KA, Manore MM, Dueck CA, Skinner JS. Disordered eating and menstrual dysfunction in female collegiate athletes. *Med Sci Sports Exerc* 1998; 30:S60.

[56] Sundgot-Borgen J. Eating disorders, energy intake, training volume, and menstrual function in high-level modern rhythmic gymnasts. *Int. J. Sport. Nutr.* 1996; 6:100-109.

[57] Weight LM, Noakes TD. Is running an analog of anorexia?: A survey of the incidence of eating disorders in female distance runners. *Med. Sci. Sports Exerc.* 1987; 19: 213-217.

[58] Ryujin DH, Breaux C, Marks AD. Symptoms of eating disorders among female distance runners: can the inconsistencies be unraveled? *Women's Health* 1999; 30: 71-83.

[59] Ashley CD, Smith JF, Robinson JB, Richardson MT. Disordered eating in female collegiate athletes and collegiate females in an advanced program of study: preliminary investigation. *Int. J. Sport. Nutr.* 1996; 6:391-401.

[60] Fogelholm M, Hiilloskorpi H. Weight and diet concerns in Finnish female and male athletes. *Med. Sci. Sports Exerc.* 1999; 31: 229-235.

[61] Hulley AJ, Hill AJ. Eating disorders and health in elite women distance runners. *Int. J. Eat. Disord.* 2002 30:312-317.

[62] Gotestam KG, Agras WS. General population-based epidemiological study of eating disorders in Norway. *Int. J. Eat. Disord.* 1995; 18:119-126.

[63] Stensland SH, Sobal J. Dietary practices of ballet, jazz, and modern dancers. *J. Am. Diet. Assoc.* 1992; 92:319-324.

[64] Beals KA. Eating behavior, nutritional status, and menstrual function in elite female adolescent volleyball players. *J. Am. Diet. Assoc.* 2002; 102:1293-1296.

[65] Beals KA. Changes in the prevalence of risk factors for the female athlete triad among collegiate athletes over a 2-year period. *Med. Sci. Sports Exerc.* 2001; 35:S285.

[66] Klungland M, Sundgot-Borgen J, Steffen K. Prevalence of the female athlete triad in Norwegian elite athletes. *Med. Sci. Sports Exerc.* 2001; 35:S227.

[67] Sundgot-Borgen J, Bahr R, Falch JA, Schneider LS. Normal bone mass in bulimic women. *J. Clin. Endocrinol.Metab.* 1998; 83:3144-3149.

[68] Rapid Weight Loss in Wrestlers Results in Death *MMWR* 47;105-108, 1998.

[69] Alderman BL, Landers DM, Carlson J, and Scott JR. Factors related to rapid weight loss practices among international-style wrestlers. *Med. Sci. Sports Exerc.* 2004; 36:249-252.

[70] Enns MP, Drewnowski A, Grinker JA. Body composition, body size estimation, and attitudes towards eating in male college athletes. *Psychosom. Med.* 1987; 49:56-64.

[71] Steen SN, Brownell KD. Patterns of weight loss and regain in wrestlers: has the tradition changed? *Med. Sci. Sports Exerc.* 1990; 22:762-768.

[72] Thiel A, Gottfried H, Hesse FW. Subclinical eating disorders in male athletes. A study of the low weight category in rowers and wrestlers. *Acta Psychiatr. Scand.* 1993; 88:259-265.

[73] Oppliger RA, Landry GL, Foster SW, Lambrecht AC. Bulimic behaviors among interscholastic wrestlers: a statewide survey. *Pediatrics* 1993; 91:826-831.

[74] Dale KS, Landers DM. Weight control in wrestling: eating disorders or disordered eating? *Med. Sci. Sports Exerc.* 1999; 31:1382-1389.

[75] Kiningham RB, Gorenflo DW. Weight loss methods of high school wrestlers. *Med. Sci. Sports Exerc.* 2001; 33: 810-813.

[76] Oppliger RA, Steen SA, Scott JR. Weight loss practices of college wrestlers. *Int. J. Sport. Nutr. Exerc. Metab.* 2003; 13:29-46.

[77] Sykora C, Grilo CM, Wilfley DE, Brownell KD. Eating, weight, and dieting disturbances in male and female lightweight and heavyweight rowers. *Int. J. Eat. Disord.* 1993; 14:203-211.

[78] Leydon MA, Wall C. New Zealond jockeys' dietary habits and their potential impact on health. *Int. J. Sport. Nutr. Exerc. Metab.* 2002; 12:220-37.

[79] Moore JM, Timperio AF, Crawford DA, Burns CM, Cameron-Smith D. Weight management and weight loss strategies of professional jockeys. *Int. J. Sport. Nutr. Exerc. Metab* 2002; 12:1-13.

[80] Parks PS, Read MH. Adolescent male athletes: body image, diet, and exercise. *Adolescence* 1997; 32:593-602.

[81] DePalma MT, Koszewski WM, Case JG, Barile RJ, DePalma BF, Oliaro SM. Weight control practices of lightweight football players. *Med. Sci. Sports Exerc.* 1993; 25:694-701.

[82] Braun DL, Sunday SR, Huang A, Halmi KA. More males seek treatment for eating disorders. *Int. J. Eat. Disord.* 1999; 25:415-24.

[83] Sherwood NE, Neumark-Sztainer D, Story M, Beuhring T, Resnick MD. Weight-related sports involvement in girls: who is at risk for disordered eating? *Am. J. Health Promot.* 2002; 16:341-344.

[84] Augestad LB, Saether B, Gotestam KG. The relationship between eating disorders and personality in physically active women. *Scand. J. Med. Sci. Sports* 1999; 9:304-12.

[85] Sundgot-Burgen J. Risk and trigger factors for the development of eating disorders in female elite athletes. *Med. Sci. Sports Exerc.* 1994; 26: 414-419.

[86] Patton GC, Johnson-Sabine E, Wood K, Mann AH, Wakeling A. Abnormal eating attitudes in London schoolgirls--a prospective epidemiological study: outcome at twelve month follow-up. *Psychol. Med.* 1990; 20:383-94.

[87] Kendler KS, MacLean C, Neale M, Kessler R, Heath A, Eaves L. The genetic epidemiology of bulimia nervosa. *Am. J. Psychiatry* 1991; 148:1627-37.

[88] Patton GC, Selzer R, Coffey C, Carlin JB, Wolfe R. Onset of adolescent eating disorders: population based cohort study over 3 years. *BMJ* 1999; 318: 765-768.

[89] Hsu, LKG. *Eating Disorders*. Guilford Press: New York, 1990.

[90] Davis C, Kennedy SH, Ravelski E, Dionne M. The role of physical activity in the development and maintenance of eating disorders. *Psychol. Med.* 1994; 24:957-67.

[91] Epling WF, Pierce WD. *Activity anorexia: Theory, research, and treatment.* Mahwah, NJ: Lawrence Erlbaum Associates, 1996.

[92] Katz JL. Long distance running, anorexia nervosa, and bulimia: a report of 2 cases. *Compr. Psychiatry* 1986; 27:74-78.

[93] Sundgot-Borgen J, Bahr R. Eating disorders in athletes. In: Harries M, ed. Oxford *Textbook of sports medicine*. New York: Oxford University Press, 1998, 138-152.

[94] Hoglund K, Normen L. A high exercise load is linked to pathological weight control behavior and eating disorders in female fitness instructors. *Scan. J. Med. Sci. Sports* 2002; 12:261-275

[95] Roberts WO, Elliot DL. Malnutrition in a compulsive runner: a case conference. *Med. Sci. Sports Exerc.* 1991; 23:513-516.

[96] O'Connor PJ, Lewis RD, Kirchner EM, Cook DB. Eating disorder symptoms in former college gymnasts: relations with body composition. *Am. J. Clin. Nutr.* 1996; 64:840-843.

[97] Yates A, Leehey K, and Shisslak C. Running—an analogue of anorexia? *N. Engl. J. Med.* 1983; 308: 251-255.

[98] Lindeman AK. Self-esteem: its application to eating disorders and athletes. *Int. J. Sport. Nutr.* 1994; 4: 237-252.

[99] Jacobi C, Hayward C, de Zwaan M, Kraemer HC, Agras WS. Coming to terms with risk factors for eating disorders: application of risk terminology and suggestions for a general taxonomy. *Psychol. Bull.* 2004; 130: 19-65.

[100] Hamilton LH, Brooks-Gunn J, Warren MP, Hamilton WG. The role of selectivity in the pathogenesis of eating problems in ballet dancers. *Med. Sci. Sports Exerc.* 1988; 20:560-565.

[101] Robinson TL, Snow-Harter C, Taaffe DR, Gillis D, Shaw J, Marcus R. Gymnasts exhibit higher bone mass than runners despite similar prevalence of amenorrhea and oligomenorrhea. *J. Bone Miner Res.* 1995;10:26-35.

[102] Helge EW, Kanstrup IL. Bone density in female elite gymnasts: impact of muscle strength and sex hormones. *Med. Sci. Sports Exerc.* 2002;34:174-180.

[103] Sudi K, Ottl K, Payerl D, Baumgartl P, Tauschmann K, Muller W. Anorexia Athletica. *Nutrition* 2004; 20: 657-661.

[104] Warren MP, Shane E, Lee MJ, Lindsay R, Dempster DW, Warren LF, Hamilton WG. Femoral head collapse associated with anorexia nervosa in a 20-year-old ballet dancer. *Clin. Orthop.* 1990; 251:171-176.

[105] Theintz G, Buchs B, Rizzoli R, Slosman D, Clavien H, Sizonenko PC, Bonjour JP. Longitudinal monitoring of bone mass accumulation in healthy adolescents: evidence for a marked reduction after 16 years of age at the levels of lumbar spine and femoral neck in female subjects. *J. Clin. Endocrinol. Metab.* 1992; 75:1060-1065.

[106] Seeman E, Szmukler GI, Formica C, Tsalamandris C, Mestrovic R. Osteoporosis in anorexia nervosa: the influence of peak bone density, bone loss, oral contraceptive use, and exercise. *J. Bone Miner. Res.* 1992; 7:1467-1474.

[107] Seeman E, Karlsson MK, Duan Y. On exposure to anorexia nervosa, the temporal variation in axial and appendicular skeletal development predisposes to site-specific deficits in bone size and density: a cross-sectional study. *J. Bone Miner. Res.* 2000; 15:2259-2265.

[108] Castro J, Lazaro L, Pons F, Halperin I, Toro J. Adolescent anorexia nervosa: the catch-up effect in bone mineral density after recovery. *J. Am. Acad. Child Adolesc. Psychiatry* 2001; 40:1215-1221.

[109] Recker RR, Davies KM, Hinders SM, Heaney RP, Stegman MR, Kimmel DB. Bone gain in young adult women. *JAMA* 1992; 268:2403-2408.

[110] Khan KM, Green RM, Saul A, Bennell KL, Crichton KJ, Hopper JL, Wark JD. Retired elite female ballet dancers and nonathletic controls have similar bone mineral density at weightbearing sites. *J. Bone Miner. Res.* 1996; 11:1556-74.

[111] Wentz E, Mellstrom D, Gillberg C, Sundh V, Gillberg IC, Rastam M. Bone density 11 years after anorexia nervosa onset in a controlled study of 39 cases. *Int. J. Eat. Disord.* 2003; 34:314-318.

[112] Jonnavithula S, Warren MP, Fox RP, Lazaro MI. Bone density is compromised in amenorrheic women despite return of menses: a 2-year study. *Obstet. Gynecol.* 1993; 81:669-674.

[113] Warren MP, Brooks-Gunn J, Fox RP, Holderness CC, Hyle EP, Hamilton WG. Osteopenia in exercise-associated amenorrhea using ballet dancers as a model: a longitudinal study. *J. Clin. Endocrinol. Metab.* 2002; 87:3162-3168.

[114] Warren MP, Brooks-Gunn J, Fox RP, Holderness CC, Hyle EP, Hamilton WG, Hamilton L. Persistent osteopenia in ballet dancers with amenorrhea and delayed menarche despite hormone therapy: a longitudinal study. *Fertil. Steril.* 2003; 80:398-404.

[115] Keen AD, Drinkwater BL. Irreversible bone loss in former amenorrheic athletes. *Osteoporos. Int.* 1997; 7:311-315.

[116] Soyka LA, Misra M, Frenchman A, Miller KK, Grinspoon S, Schoenfeld DA, Klibanski A. Abnormal bone mineral accrual in adolescent girls with anorexia nervosa. *J. Clin. Endocrinol. Metab.* 2002; 87:4177-4185.

[117] Vestergaard P, Emborg C, Stoving RK, Hagen C, Mosekilde L, Brixen K. Fractures in patients with anorexia nervosa, bulimia nervosa, and other eating disorders—a nationwide register study. *Int. J. Eat. Disord.* 2002; 32: 301-308.

[118] Vestergaard P, Emborg C, Stoving RK, Hagen C, Mosekilde L, Brixen K. Patients with eating disorders. A high-risk group for fractures. *Orthop. Nurs.* 2003;22:325-331.

[119] Rigotti NA, Neer RM, Skates SJ, Herzog DB, Nussbaum SR. The clinical course of osteoproris in anorexia nervosa. *JAMA* 1991; 265: 1133.

[120] Lucas AR, Melton LJ, Crowson CS, O'Fallon WM. Long-term fracture risk among women with anorexia nervosa: a population-based cohort study. *Mayo Clin. Proc.*1999; 74:972-977.

[121] Kontulainen S, Sievanen H, Kannus P, Pasanen M, Vuori I. Effect of long-term impact-loading on mass, size, and estimated strength of humerus and radius of female racquet-sports players: a peripheral quantitative computed tomography study between young and old starters and controls. *J. Bone Miner. Res.* 2003; 18:352-359.

[122] Bass S, Bradney M, Pearce G, Hendrich E, Inge K, Stuckey S, Lo SK, Seeman E. Short stature and delayed puberty in gymnasts: influence of selection bias on leg length and the duration of training on trunk length. *J. Pediatr.* 2000; 136:149-155.

[123] Caine D, Lewis R, O'Connor P, Howe W, Bass S. Does gymnastics training inhibit growth of females? *Clin. J. Sport. Med.*2001; 11:260-270.

[124] Andersen AE, Watson T, Schlechte J. Osteoporosis and osteopenia in men with eating disorders. *Lancet* 2000; 355:1967-1968.

[125] Thienpont E, Bellemans J, Samson I, Fabry G. Stress fracture of the inferior and superior pubic ramus in a man with anorexia nervosa and hypogonadism. *Acta Orthop. Belg.* 2000; 66:297-301.

[126] Myers S, Bell D, Gorman J, Best J, Rooney J. Repetition of an unusual stress fracture in an anorexic man: a case report. *J. Orthop. Surg.* 2002; 10:210-212.

[127] Bilanin JE, Blanchard MS, Russek-Cohen E. Lower vertebral bone density in male long distance runners. *Med. Sci. Sports Exerc.* 1989; 21:66-70.

[128] Hetland ML, Haarbo J, Christiansen C. Low bone mass and high bone turnover in male long distance runners. *J. Clin. Endocrinol. Metab.* 1993; 77:770-775.

[129] Warren MP, Brooks-Gunn J, Hamilton LH, Warren LF, Hamilton WG. Scoliosis and fractures in young ballet dancers. Relation to delayed menarche and secondary amenorrhea. *N. Engl. J. Med.* 1986; 315:905.

[130] Barrow GW, Saha S. Menstrual irregularity and stress fractures in collegiate female distance runners. *Am. J. Sports Med.* 1988;16: 209-216.

[131] Beckvid HG, Schnell C, Linden HA. Women endurance runners with menstrual dysfunction have prolonged interruption of training due to injury. *Gynecol. Obstet. Invest.* 2000; 49: 41-46.

[132] Fogelholm M. Effects of bodyweight reduction on sports performance. *Sports Med.* 1994; 18: 249-267.

[133] Webster S, Rutt R, Weltman A. Physiological effects of a weight loss regimen practiced by college wrestlers. *Med. Sci. Sports Exerc.* 1990; 22: 229-234.

[134] Horswill CA. Weight loss and weight cycling in amateur wrestlers: implications for performance and resting metabolic rate. *Int. J. Sport Nutr.* 1993; 3:245-260.

[135] Roemmich JN, Sinning WE. Weight loss and wrestling training: effects on nutrition, growth, maturation, body composition, and strength. *J. Appl. Physiol.* 1997; 82:1751-1759.

[136] Crow S, Praus B, Thuras P. Mortality from eating disorders—a 5- to 10-year record linkage study. *Int. J. Eat. Disord.* 1999; 26: 97-101.

[137] Ratnasuriya RH, Eisler I, Szmukler GI, Russell GF. Anorexia Nervosa: Outcome and prognostic factors after 20 years. *Br. J. Psychiatry* 1991; 158:495-502.

[138] Iacovino JR. Anorexia nervosa: a 63-year population-based survival study. *J. Insur. Med.* 2004; 36:107-110.

[139] Holderness CC, Brooks-Gunn J, Warren MP. Eating disorders and substance use: a dancing vs. a nondancing population. *Med. Sci. Sports Exerc.* 1994; 26:297-302.

[140] Sanchez-Cardenas M, Paruit Portes C. Eating disorders and suicide attempts in 2 dance students. *Arch. Pediatr.* 1996; 3:51-54.

[141] Gutgesell ME, Timmerman MG. Alcohol use and behaviors in women long-distance race participants reporting a history of bulimia and/or anorexia nervosa. *J. Sports Med. Phys. Fitness* 1998; 38: 142-148.

[142] Misra M and Klibanski A. Evaluation and treatment of low bone density in anorexia nervosa. *Nutr. Clin. Care* 2002; 5: 293-308.

[143] Vohs KD, Heatherton TF, Herrin M. Disordered eating and the transition to college: a prospective study. *Int. J. Eat. Disord.* 2001; 29: 280-288.

[144] Beals KA. Eating disorder and menstrual dysfunction screening, education, and treatment programs. *Phys. Sportsmed.* 1993; 31.

[145] Vaughan JL, King KA, Cottrell RR. Collegiate athletic trainers'confidence in helping female athletes with eating disorders. *J. Athl. Train.* 2004; 39:71-76.

[146] Rumball JS, Lebrun CM. Preparticipation physical examination: selected issues for the female athlete. *Clin. J. Sport. Med.* 2004; 14:153-60.

[147] Carek PJ, Futrell M. Athletes' view of the preparticipation physical examination. Attitudes toward certain health screening questions. *Arch. Fam. Med.* 1999; 8:307-312.

[148] Juzwiak CR, Ancona-Lopez F. Evaluation of nutrition knowledge and dietary recommendations by coaches of adolescent Brazilian athletes. *Int. J. Sport. Nutr. Metab.* 2004; 14: 222-235.

[149] Deutz RC, Benardot D, Martin DE, Cody MM. Relationship between energy deficits and body composition in elite female gymnasts and runners. *Med Sci Sports Exerc* 2000; 32:659-668.

[150] Judex S and Zernicke RF. High impact exercise and growing bone: relation between high strain rates and enhanced bone formation. *J. Appl. Physiol.* 2000; 88:2183-2191.

[151] Fuchs RK, Bauer JJ, Snow CM. Jumping improves hip and lumbar spine bone mass in prepubescent children: a randomized controlled trial. *J. Bone. Miner. Res.* 2001; 16:148-56.

[152] Heinonen A, Sievanen H, Kannus P, Oja P, Pasanen M, Vouri I. High-impact exercise and bones of growing girls: a 9-month controlled trial. *Osteoporos. Int.* 2000; 11:1010-1017.

[153] Taaffe DR, Robinson TL, Snow CM, Marcus R. High-impact exercise promotes bone gain in well-trained female athletes. *J. Bone Miner. Res.* 1997; 12:255-260.

[154] Morris FL, Payne WR, Wark JD. The impact of intense training on endogenous estrogens and progesterone concentrations and bone mineral acquisition in adolescent rowers. *Osteoporos Int.* 1999; 10:361-368.

[155] Milgrom C, Simkin A, Eldad A, Nyska M, Finestone A. Using bone's adaptation ability to lower the incidence of stress fractures. *Am. J. Sports Med.* 2000; 28:245-251.

[156] Bass S, Pearce G, Bradney M, Hendrich E, Delmas PD, Harding A, Seeman E. Exercise before puberty may confer residual benefits in bone density in adulthood: studies in active prepubertal and retired female gymnasts. *J. Bone Miner. Res.* 1998; 13:500-507.

[157] Joy E, Clark N, Ireland ML, Martire J, Nattiv A, Varechok S. Team management of the female athlete triad: Part 2: Optimal treatment and prevention tactics. *Physician Sportsmed.* 1997; 25.

[158] Braam LA, Knapen MH, Geusens P, Brouns F, Vermeer C. Factors affecting bone loss in female endurance athletes: a two-year follow-up study. *Am. J. Sports. Med.* 2003; 31:889-895.

[159] Rickenlund A, Carlstrom K, Ekblom B, Brismar TB, Von Schoultz B, Hirschberg AL. Effects of oral contraceptives on body composition and physical performance in female athletes. *J. Clin. Endocrinol. Metab.* 2000; 89:4364-4370.

[160] Cumming DC. Exercise-associated amenorrhea, low bone density, and estrogen replacement therapy. *Arch. Intern. Med.* 1996; 156:2193-2195.

[161] Golden NH, Lanzkowsky L, Schebendach J, Palestro CJ, Jacobson MS, Shenker IR. The effect of estrogen-progestin treatment on bone mineral density in anorexia nervosa. *J. Pediatr. Adolesc. Gynecol.* 2002; 15:135-143.

[162] Munoz MT, Morande G, Garcia-Centenera JA, Hervas F, Pozo J, Argente J. The effects of estrogen administration on bone mineral density in adolescents with anorexia nervosa. *Eur. J. Endocrinol.* 2002; 146:45-50.

[163] Gibson JH, Mitchell A, Reeve J, Harries MG. Treatment of reduced bone mineral density in athletic amenorrhea: a pilot study. *Osteoporos. Int.* 1999; 10:284-289.

[164] Klibanski A, Biller BM, Schoenfeld DA, Herzog DB, Sace VC. The effects of estrogen administration on trabecular bone loss in young women with anorexia nervosa. *J. Clin. Endocrinol. Metab.* 1995; 80:898-904.

[165] Grinspoon S, Thomas L, Miller K, Herzog D, Klibanski A. Effects of recombinant human IGF-I and oral contraceptive administration on bone density in anorexia nervosa. *J. Clin. Endrocrinol.* Metab. 2002; 87:2883-2891.

[166] Robinson E, Bachrach LK, Katzman DK. Use of hormone replacement therapy to reduce the risk of osteopenia in adolescent girls with anorexia nervosa. *J. Adoles. Health* 2000; 26:343.

[167] Jamieson MA, Katzman DK, Cromer B. Hormone replacement in the adolescent with anorexia and hypothalmic amenorrhea—yes or no? *J Pediatr Adolesc Gynecol* 2001; 14:39-45.

[168] Harel Z, Riggs S. Transdermal versus oral administration of estrogen in the management of lumbar spine osteopenia in an adolescent with anorexia nervosa. *J. Adol. Health*.1997; 21:179-182.

[169] Haberland CA, Seddick D, Marcus R, Bachrach LK. A physician survey of therapy for exercise-associated amenorrhea: a brief report. *Clin. J. Sport Med.* 1995; 5:246-250.

[170] Gordon CM, Grace E, Emans SJ, Feldman HA, Goodman E, Becker KA, Rosen CJ, Gundberg CM, LeBoff MS. Effects of oral dehydroepiandrosterone on bone density in young women with anorexia nervosa: a randomized trial. *J. Clin. Endocrinol. Metab.* 2002; 87:4935-41.

[171] Welt CK, Chan JL, Bullen J, Murphy R, Smith P, DePaoli AM, Karalis A, Mantzoros CS. Recombinant human leptin in women with hypothalamic amenorrhea. *N. Engl. J. Med.* 2004; 351:987-997.

[172] Miller KK, Grieco KA, Mulder J, Grinspoon S, Mickley D, Yehezkel R, Herzog DB, Klibanski A. Effect of risedronate on bone density in anorexia nervosa. *J. Clin. Endricronol. Metab.* 2004; 89:3903-3906.

[173] Marini JC. Do bisphosphonates make children's bones better or brittle? *N. Engl. J. Med.* 2003; 349:423-426.

In: Hot Topics in Sports and Athletics
Editor: Samuel R. Bakere, pp. 51-59
ISBN 978-1-60456-077-0

Chapter 3

Buyer Satisfaction, Purchasing Decision and Relative Contribution of Promotion Tools for Olympic Products: The ATHENS 2004 Experience

Despina Karayianni [1] ***and John Mylonakis*** [2]
University of Patra, Department of Business Administration,
Panepistimioupoli, Rio, 26500, Patra, Greece

Abstract

The chapter intends to examine the consumer attitude towards ATHENS 2004 Olympic Products, their purchasing behavior, as well as, the impact of the various means of promotion on their attitude and purchasing behavior. ATHENS 2004 Olympic Products are more than simple souvenir products. They bear the ATHENS 2004 emblem and its characteristics, representing the visual identity of the ATHENS 2004 Olympic Games The research results lead to certain useful conclusions on Sports Marketing, which may be used either by existing sports organizations with their organized marketing departments or on future large-scale sports events, such as the Beijing 2008 Olympic Games.

Keywords: *Olympic Games, Olympic Products, Sports Marketing, Consumer Behavior*

---

[1] E-mail: karayan@otenet.gr.
[2] 10 Nikiforou Str., Glyfada, 166 75, Athens, Greece, E-mail: imylonakis@panafonet.gr.

1. Introduction

Over the last years, Sports Marketing has received increased attention from academics and professionals. It is now accepted into the generic framework of Marketing of Services, acknowledging the unique features of sport services products and the environment in which they are produced (Westrbeek and Shilbury, 2003). Customers buy sports offerings consisting of goods, services, information, personal attention and other components.

According to the fundamental principles of the Olympic Spirit (or Olympism) aims to contribute to a peaceful and better world by educating youth through sport practiced without discrimination of any kind (Olympic Charter, 2001). Olympic Games are a universal concept, having become one of the most popular, most watched, large-scale and profitable global events. Thus, all visitors and spectators become interconnected parts among the diverse cultures of the world (Hunterformer, 2001), which organizers must understand, respect and demonstrate (Trompenaars and Woolliams, 2004).

Olympic licensing programs are targeted to market officially licensed products and merchandise from the Olympic family (Organizing Committee, National Committee, and International Olympic Committee). Visitors buy and consume Olympic souvenirs and goods with Olympic logos and symbols that will remind them of the games and organizing city. Many global companies spend huge amounts on sponsoring their brands in order to capitalize on the Olympic Games' image.

ATHENS 2004 Olympic Products were more than simple souvenir products. They bore the ATHENS 2004 emblem and its characteristics, representing the visual identity of the ATHENS 2004 Olympic Games. They expressed the return of the Games to their country of origin and communicate their timeless values. Friendship, Moral, fair Play and Participation all become a philosophy and an expression of life before, after and during the Games. Thus, the aim of the present paper was to analyze the attitude of consumers' attitude towards Olympic Products along with the factors affecting purchasing decision and consumer satisfaction.

Previous Sport marketing research has focused on different marketing issues like, sport services quality principles (Chang et al., 2002), sport services values and satisfaction (Westerbeek and Shilbury, 2003), marketing and promotion of Olympic Games (Lee, 2005), as well as, sport consumption (Funk, 2002) and the influences on the host city (Mueller et al., 2006, Kartakoulis et al., 2003, Green, 2002, Woodside et al., 2002, Ratnatunga and Mt Eliza, 2000) and the consumer (Roy and Graeff, 2003) advertisement and networks, promotion and sponsorship techniques and its globalization effects (Jackson, 2000). Research regarding how customers perceive the value of sports goods and services and what benefits they are looking for has, also, been cited (Papadimitriou et al., 2004, Mitchell et al., 2004, d' Astous and Chnaoui, 2002). Despite the aforementioned findings Marketing Research on the role of product, price and intended usage situation on Olympic products seems to have fallen behind. The pioneering contribution of this research is that it pays special attention to the specific examination of the consumers' perception and responses to Olympic apparels.

The Beijing Organizing Committee for the Games has urged consumers to buy Olympic products from licensed stores in order to avoid purchasing counterfeit goods. It has licensed

2000 items of Olympic products, including casual cloths, pins and sports equipment (Beijing 2008).

2. Research Methodology

In order to reach the above aim, we followed the steps of scientific methodology of research, as described below. This study is divided into three stages. The first two stages refer to the collection of data and the third to statistical analysis. More specifically:

A thorough preliminary study was initially conducted, including:

- Review on related literature to Olympic Products, consumer attitude and behavior, brand value (Olympic Products brand) and the means of consumer products promotion (Siomkos, 2002, Bearden et al., 1989), and
- Primary qualitative research based on an unstructured questionnaire (open questions) and thorough interviews with 35 selected Olympic Products buyers, in order to determine the criteria forming prospective buyer expectations for the examined products.

Based on the existing literature review, as well as, on the findings of the preliminary qualitative research we compiled a questionnaire used the second and main stage. In order to measure the attitude of Olympic Products consumers, 5-level Likert scales were used (I strongly agree=5, I strongly disagree=10. On questions referring to the reasons for purchase and the types of Olympic Products, hierarchical scales of preferences were used, while for the information sources of the answers (promotion data), the points of sale and the demographic data we used dichotomous questions (Stathakopoulos, 2000).

The second stage of data collection was based on a structured questionnaire and refers to the quantitative market research, conducted in three days and involving personal interviews with citizens passing from central points in the cities of Athens and Patra. Overall, 170 people participated in this research, 95 from Athens and 75 from the city of Patra.

The third stage involves a series of detailed statistical analyses of data, from which findings emerge and lead to several conclusions. These conclusions are of use to the marketing executives of sports organizations and the organizers of large sports events.

3. Research Findings

Sample Description

In the research 90 men and 80 women consumers participated, representing 57% and 43% of the sample, respectively. Of them 63% are 18-29 years of age while the remaining 27% of the sample is 30-50 years of age. Moreover, 34% of the participants' declaration of income is up to 600 euros, while 60% declared income above 600 euros. In terms of occupation, 35% of the sample are students, 17% are civil servants and the remaining 48% work in the private sector.

It should be mentioned that the results of this research did not present any statistical important differences on questions regarding demographic elements, apart from the area where the research was conducted. This allows us to consider the sample as homogenous and to include all sample data in our statistical analysis. Differences due to the location of the research are shown below.

Attitudes and Purchasing Behavior

Out of 170 participants, only 49 persons claimed to have purchased an Olympic product, corresponding to 29% of the total sample. The following table shows the attitude of Olympic Products buyers included in the sample, as emerges from the average values of their purchasing criteria.

Table 1. Consumer Expectations on Olympic Products

	Average	Std. Dev.
Olympic Products have a nice appearance	4.25	8.9
It is worth giving an Olympic Product as gift to friends/relatives	4.25	1.1
Olympic Products are made of excellent quality materials	3.85	8.9
I can easily find a store selling Olympic Products	3.80	1.2
Olympic Products store employees are very helping	3.70	1.2
Olympic Products value for money is acceptable	2.90	1.1

As was expected, there is a difference in attitudes towards Olympic Products between buyers and non-buyers. These differences are shown in Table 2.

Table 2. Different Attitudes among Olympic Products' Buyers and Non-buyers

Average Buyers Non-Buyers		
Olympic Products have a nice appearance	4.25	3.80
It is worth giving an Olympic Product as gift to friends/relatives	4.25	3.78
Olympic Products are made of excellent quality materials	3.85	3.36
Olympic Products store employees are very helping	3.70	3.30

From Tables 1 and 2 it emerges that nearly all variables used as criteria forming buyer attitude constitute determinant factors of purchasing behavior (the most important distinction between buyers and non-buyers).

Further, the above set of questions was examined as a single variable, the Olympic Products buyer satisfaction, following bibliographical directions regarding satisfaction after purchase and market research (Parasuraman et al., 1988; Churchill, 2000). More specifically, the above 6 elements were subject to reliability analysis, the statistical result of which was above the allowed limit (Coefficient alpha= .73). This fact allowed us to add up all constituent elements.

The average of this aggregated variable presents a statistically significant difference between buyers (3.85) and non-buyers (3.86), a fact that highlights the validity of the scale (since satisfaction mainly derives from post-purchase experience). Moreover, the average of this variable did not present any statistically significant differences in relation to the sample's demographic elements.

Sources of Information

Table 3 shows the hierarchical percentages of information sources for the whole sample. The study revealed that a statistically significant percentage of non-buyers (79%) have been informed about the Olympic Products through television. A statistically large percentage of non-buyers claimed that they have not been informed by friends or acquaintances. These findings combined demonstrate that Olympic Products' promotion, at least as performed in spring 2003, is largely related to Olympic Products sales, while the opposite stands for recommendations by friends or relatives. A strong relation also exists between Olympic Products' promotion by celebrities and Olympic Products purchasing decision by consumers (3.9 against 3.7 for non-buyers, respectively), thus verifying all relevant literature data (Reynolds and Darden, 1971).

Table 3. Sources of Information on Olympic Products

%	
Television	38.0
Magazine/Newspaper	17.0
Friends/Acquaintances	17.0
Radio	5.0
Other Sources	4.0
Internet	3.0

The above findings lead to further analysis and results:

Substantial differences exist in the average of the *Satisfaction by Olympic Products appearance* variable in relation to TV promotion. More specifically, those informed by TV were less satisfied by Olympic Products appearance (4.2 against 3.6). On the other hand, those informed by friends and acquaintances were much more satisfied with Olympic Products quality (7.7 against 3.4) and appearance (4.3 against 3.7), compared to the rest.

Overall, the above results demonstrate a rather inadequate promotion through television, a fact that discourages purchase and is due to further study (Mehta, 2000). Also, positive word-of-mouth communication has influenced the decision of purchase, a fact that increases

Olympic Products quality and is confirmed by international bibliography (Flynn, et al., 1996; McGuire, 1968; Bearden et al., 1989).

Points of Sale

As shown in Table 4, the most preferred point of sale is the Internet, followed by authorized Olympic Products stores, the airport and post offices. It is worth mentioning that Olympic booths are ranked as last in the preferences of buyers among the other available points of sale (it is possible that, at the time this study took place, the location of these booths was not widely known). Department stores were, also, less favored by consumers, possibly due to the fact that Olympic Products are considered to be of high quality, thus must be sold in more specialized stores (Siomkos, 2002).

Table 4. Olympic Products Points of Sale

Average Std. Dev.		
Internet	5.07	1.4
Other Stores	4.23	1.4
Airport	3.84	1.3
Post Office	3.61	1.5
Department Store	2.26	1.1
Olympic Store	1.99	1.2

Local Differences

The study revealed certain differences in the market ratio and types of Olympic Products between Athens and the countryside. More particularly, Athens citizens would buy Olympic Products for their historical value (claiming that they would add them to their personal collection), while citizens of Patra would rather offer them as a gift to friends and relatives. Also, Athens citizens would prefer an Olympic pin, while Patra citizens chose a mug. Moreover, people living in the countryside appear to be better informed, not only through television (72% against 44.4%) but also through the printer media (36% against 18%), compared to people living in Athens.

4. Conclusion

In this paper we present the results of an exploratory research which attempts to examine the level of consumer attitude as well as buyer satisfaction from Olympic Products. The relationship between the various sources of information and the decision for purchase are also considered. The findings lead to certain remarkable results.

The variables used to measure buyer satisfaction by Olympic Products were valid and reliable. Olympic Products buyers claimed that they were satisfied with product quality. Even though television was the primary source of information on Olympic Products, the image it created was not satisfactory; contrary to general belief television showed a negative impact on consumer purchasing decision.

Friends and relatives were the second cited source of information (along with the magazines and newspapers). Friends and relatives showed a positive impact on consumer satisfaction in terms of Olympic Products appearance and quality (e.g. positive recommendations made by buyers to new prospective buyers).

The study also revealed certain cultural differences among the various geographical areas, demonstrating that people residing in the Capital showed a more atomistic behavior compared to people residing in the countryside who showed a rather socially-motivated behavior when buying Olympic Products.

Olympic Games organization has become part of our society's fabric; they offer the chance to reconcile cultures, to bridge social and economic gaps and to improve the quality of life for billion of visitors, spectators and consumers; they also provide an opportunity for global business, as well as, international and local organizations to offer differentiated products and services.

It seems that in the case of Olympic Products the expensive above the line promotion tools (i.e. TV promotion) seems to be less effective in gaining consumer satisfaction than below the line promotion counterparts (i.e. word of mouth communication). Future organizers of international and local sport events should take the above findings into consideration in order to organize more effective promotion strategies.

Furthermore, they should, also, focus on regional differences (i.e. behavioural differences among consumers residing in the capital versus countryside). Regional differences should, also, focus on the idiosyncratic characteristics of the targeted consumer per se. The research also revealed some interesting regional differences in respect to sources of information and purchase motives between residents of the capital and the countryside. However, these last issues need more extensive research.

References

Beaden, W., Netemeyer, R., Teel J., (1989), "Measurement of consumer susceptibility to interpersonal influence", *Journal of Consumer Research*, 15, 4, pp. 473-481.

Beijing 2008 Olympic Games, "Consumers advised to buy Olympic products from licensed stores", available at http://en.beijing2008.com - 13 Dec. 2006.

Chang, C-M., Chen, C-T., Hsu, C-H, (2002), "A Review of Service Quality in Corporate and Recreational Sport/Fitness Programs", *The Sport Journal,* Spring, Vol. 5, No. 3.

Churchill, G., (2000), *"Marketing Research, Methodological Foundations"*, Irwin D' Astous , A., Chnaoui, K., (2002),"Consumer perception of sports apparel: the role of brand name, store name, price and intended usage situation", June/July, Vol. 4, No. 2.

Flyn, R.L., Goldsmith, G., Eastman, J.K., (1996), "Opinion Leaders and Opinion Seekers", *Journal of Marketing*, 12, p. 26.

Funk, D., (2002), "Consumer-Based Marketing: The Use of Micro-Segmentation Strategies for Understanding Sport Consumption", *International Journal of Sports Marketing and Sponsorship*, September/October, Vol. 4, No. 3 .

Hunterformer, D. (2001), "Olympism for the 21st Century: New Life to a Timeless Philosophy, *The Sport Journal,* Spring, Vol. 4, No. 1.

Jackson, S. (2000), "Sports Marketing and the Challenges of Globalization: A Case Study of Cultural Resistance in New Zealand", *International Journal of Sports Marketing and Sponsorship*, June/July, Vol. 2, No. 2 .

Kartakoulis, N., Papanikos, G., Karlis, G., (2003), "City and Sport Marketing Strategy: The Case of Athens 2004", *The Sport Journal*, Spring, Vol. 6, No. 2.

Lee, J. (2005), "Marketing and Promotion of the Olympic Games", *The Sport Journal*, Vol. 8, No. 3.

McGuire, W., (1968), "Personality and Susceptibility to Social Influence", in *Handbook of personality Theory and Research*, Edgar F. Borgatta and W. Lamberts (eds), Chicago, pp. 1130-1187.

Mehta, A., (2000), "Advertising Attitudes and Advertising Effectiveness", *Journal of Advertising Research*, 40,3, pp.67-72

Mitchell, M., Montgomery R., Mitchell, S., (2004), "Consumer Experience Tourism and Brand Bonding: A Look at Sport-Related Marketers", *The Sport Journal,* Vol. 7, No. 2.

Mueller, N., Messing, M., Preus, H., Desh, M., Buchwalder, M., (2006), *The Sport Journal*, Vol. 9, No. 1.

Olympic Charter (2001), "The Fundamental Principles of Olympism", *The Sport Journal*, Vol. 4, No. 1.

Papadimitriou, D., Apostolopoulou, A., Loukas, I., (2004), "The role of perceived fit in fans' evaluation of sports brand extension", *International Journal of Sports Marketing and Sponsorship,* July, Vol. 6, No. 1 .

Parasuraman, A., Zeithaml, V. A., and Berry, L. L., (1988), "SERVQUAL: A Multiple-Item Scale for Measuring Consumer Perceptions of Service Quality", *Journal of Retailing*, 64, pp. 12-40.

Ratnatunga, J., Mt Eliza, M., (2000), "Lessons from Atlanta Olympics: marketing and organizational considerations for Sydney 2000", *International Journal of Sports Marketing and Sponsorship*, September/October, Vol. 2, No. 3 .

Reynolds, F., Darden, W. (1971), "Mutually Adaptive Effects of Interpersonal Communications", *Journal of Marketing Research*, No. 8 .

Roy, D. and Graeff, T., (2003), "Influences on Consumer Responses to Winter Olympic Sponsorship", International *Journal of Sports Marketing and Sponsorship*, December/January, Vol. 3, No. 4.

Siomkos, G., (2000), Consumer Behaviour", Stamoulis Publications, Athens.

Stathakopoulos, V., (2000), "*Market Research Methods*", Stamoulis Publications, Athens.

Trompenhaars, F., Woolliams P., (2004), "*Marketing Across Cultures*", Capstone, pp. 16-17.

Westerbeek, H. and Shilbury, D. (2003), "A conceptual model for sport services marketing research: integrating quality, value and satisfaction", *International Journal of Sports Marketing and Sponsorship,* March/April, Vol. 5, No. 1.

Woodside, A., Spurr, R., March, R., Clark, H. (2002), "The Dynamics of Traveler Destination Awareness and Search for Information Associated with Hosting the Olympic Games", *International Journal of Sports Marketing and Sponsorship*, June/July, Vol. 4, No 2 .

Biographical Notes

Dr. Despina Karayianni is Assistant Professor of Marketing at the Business Administration Department of the University of Patra. She holds a Ph.D in Marketing, an M.B.A. and a B.A. in Business Administration from the Athens Economic University. Her interests are in Relations and Interactive Marketing. She has published several papers regarding Business Networking and Internet Marketing in academic journals and has participated in many international conferences.

Dr. John Mylonakis is currently Tutor at the Hellenic Open University. He was Visiting Professor of Marketing at the Vrije Universiteit, Bruxelles and the Institute Catholique des Haute Etudes Commerciales, as well as, Board Member of the International Board of Auditors at NATO in Brussels, Belgium. He holds a BA in Business Administration, a M.Sc. in International Business and a Ph.D. in Marketing of Financial Services. He has taught for over 20 years at several Universities in Greece and Belgium. He has published several papers in academic journals and articles in professional editions and has participated in many international conferences. He is, also, Editorial Board member for several international academic journals.

In: Hot Topics in Sports and Athletics
Editor: Samuel R. Bakere, pp. 61-77
ISBN 978-1-60456-077-0

Chapter 4

Can Spectators' Mood Be Manipulated and Maintained in a Losing Game?: Interaction between Team Identification and Pre-Game Mood

Hyungil Harry Kwon*[3], *Chulwon Lee and Sang-il Lee
Florida State University,USA
Yonsei Univeristy, China
Sookmyung Women's Univeristy,China

Abstract

The current study addressed two research questions. First, study 1 examined whether spectators' mood before they were exposed to a losing game (i.e., pre-game mood) influenced their mood after the game (post-game mood) and their information processing. Secondly, study 2 examined whether the influence of pre-game mood found in Study 1 was modified by personal relevance (i.e., team identification) with a sporting game. The results indicated that pre-game mood influenced participants' post-game mood and information processing system. The results of the second study also supported the hypotheses that post-game mood and spectators' information processing were influenced by pre-game mood and personal relevance (i.e., team identification). As hypothesized, two-way interaction between pre-game mood and personal relevance was found in post-game mood whereas no interaction was found in information processing. This study was able to identify a group of people who were more affected by the result of home game and who were more effectively responded to mood manipulation.

3 Correspondence concerning this article should be addressed to Dr. Hyungil Harry Kwon, Assistant Professor, Sport Management, Recreation Management, and Physical Education Department, Florida State University, 120A Tully Gym. P. O. Box 4280. Tallahassee, FL 32306-4280. Phone # (850) 645-2350. Fax (850) 644-0975. Electronic mail may be sent via Internet to kwon@coe.fsu.edu.

Introduction

Marketing scholars and practitioners have been interested in how consumers react to a product trial. In particular, a large body of literature is available in service marketing in relation to customer satisfaction (Alford and Sherrell, 1996; Dube and Menon, 2000; Lijander and Strandvik, 1997; Oliver, 1997). In many different service industries, the causal relationship among affective state of customers, satisfaction, and behavioral intention (e.g., future repatronage) has been found and confirmed repeatedly. In spectating sport service, the relationship between post-game affective state (e.g., enjoyment) and future fan behaviors (e.g., future game attendance, licensed merchandise purchase) has been confirmed through confirmatory manner such as structural equation modeling (i.e., Madrigal, 1995; Trail, Fink, and Anderson, 2003).

However, knowing that sport marketers have no control over the performance of a sporting game (i.e., sport marketers cannot guarantee spectators having positive affect after a sporting game), a confirmation of the positive causal relationship between affective state after a game and future repatronage has little practical value to sport marketers. Thus, a line of research regarding how to influence and manipulate the post-game affective state of spectators is necessary for aforementioned relationship to have a practical value.

The current study, through two experimental studies, attempted to see whether an affective state of spectators (i. e., mood) can be manipulated, by management, to an extent that they feel less negatively after they watch a losing home game. The first study examined whether a manipulated positive mood can be maintained even after participants had negative product trial (i.e., watching a losing game of a home team) and whether this causes different type of information processing (i.e., amount of cognitive elaboration). The second study attempted to examine the effect of mood state and personal relevance (i.e., team identification) before a product trial on the evaluation of a negative product trial (i.e., a losing game). The second study also examined whether the effect of pre-game mood was modified by personal relevance (i.e., team identification). The ultimate objective of the two studies is to identify the characteristics of the spectators (i.e., in terms of the team identification) who are more susceptible to negative game outcome and mood manipulation. Sport marketers, with this information in their hands, can identify a group of spectators whose negative feeling actually can be remedied, to a certain extent, by receiving any incentive that makes them happy. The study is based on dual information processing (Chaiken, Giner-Sorolla, and Chen, 1996), elaboration likelihood model (ELM, Petty and Cacioppo, 1986), and affect infusion model (AIM, Forgas, 1995) as its theoretical bases.

Study 1

Sport Consumers and Game Outcome

Sport spectators' affective state is largely determined by the results of a game (Trail, Fink, and Anderson, 2003). Empirical supports can be found in Madrigal (1995) and Trail, Fink, and Anderson (2003). Madrigal (1995) developed the Model of Fan Satisfaction, in which a causal relationship between expectancy confirmation (i.e., win or loss) and enjoyment was hypothesized and confirmed. Trail, Fink, and Anderson (2003) also confirmed a causal relationship between expectancies (dis) confirmation and affective state. Further influence of affective state after a game on satisfaction (Madrigal, 1995) and future fan behavior (Trail et al., 2003) were also confirmed in the literature. Spectators with positive affective state after a confirmation of expectancy are expected to have a positive affective state (e.g., happy) and it leads to customer satisfaction and more repatronage in terms of game attendance and licensed merchandise sales.

The causal relationship between game results, affective state, satisfaction, and future fan behavior provided a marketing implication that sport teams need to win every game or, at least, perform well up to the expectation of customers to make them happy, which is quite impossible. For this reason, frameworks in affect and information processing were explored to see whether affective state (e.g., mood) of spectators can be manipulated and maintained using non-performance related variables in spectating sport environment. Among those, major thesis of the current study is based on the evidence that mood of people can be maintained (e.g., Handley, Lassiter, Nickell, and Herchenroeder, 2004; Isen and Patrick, 1983; Isen and Simmonds, 1978).

Mood and Its Maintenance

People in positive mood perceive things in a more positive way (Bower, 1981; Carlson and Adams, 1980; Clark and Teasdale, 1985; Forgas, Bower, and Krantz, 1984; Isen, Shalker, Clark, and Karp, 1978). This process of *priming* puts oneself in a loop of positive thinking. Thus, people in a positive mood evaluate an event more positively than people in neutral or negative mood (Clark and Isen, 1982). The maintenance of the mood depends on how long and how intensively a person can stay in the loop of positive thinking. It is obvious that people can stay longer in a positive mood if he/she experiences more subsequent happy events. The people in positive mood try to engage themselves in a happy situation (e.g., helping others) so that they can extend the time period of being in positive mood (Isen and Simmonds, 1978).

Isen, Clark and Schwartz (1976) examined the duration of the effect of a good mood. Their experiment started with mood manipulation; the positive mood was manipulated by giving away a free sample of stationery, which was about 20 cents worth. The participants were divided into two groups; the ones who received the free stationary and the ones who did not receive anything. All the participants received wrong number phone calls during which they could provide help to the caller. They counted the number of subjects who helped and who did not help to determine group differences. Measuring the percentage of subjects who helped in different time after receiving the incentive, the researchers found that participants in the treatment group (i.e., free stationary) helped more than the participants in the control group (i.e., no incentive). They also found that the effect diminished gradually over time; the two groups showed no difference after 20 minutes. The results indicated that the percentage of who helped was greatest in the five minutes condition (100%), while the percentage gradually declined to the same level (10%) as the control group after 20 minutes.

Another line of research proposed the same mood maintenance mechanism with the emphasis on information processing. This line of research focuses on how people process incoming information in different mood states. Chaiken et al. (1996) argued that people in a positive mood incorporated rapid and less effortful strategies in solving a problem. People want to prolong their positive mood by disengaging themselves from processing any negative information (Batra and Stephens, 1994). This phenomenon was clearly detected in Isen and Simmonds' (1978) study, in which people in good mood were more likely to help someone if the helping tasking is reading pleasant information but help less if the information is negative. Based on the previous literature it can be conjectured that people in positive mood actively protect the current good mood by engaging themselves in pleasant events or by blocking themselves from negative information. Thus, it is cautiously speculated that if spectators are manipulated to be in a positive mood, they may try to maintain the positive mood and show a better mood after they watch a losing game than the ones who are not manipulated to be in a positive mood. The losing game can provide many different types of negative information to the spectators (e.g., bad formation, bad strategies, bad call, etc.). However, the ones in a positive mood will be blocking negative incoming information more than the ones in a neutral or negative mood. Based on this theorizing, a hypothesis was generated as below.

Hypothesis 1:

Participants in a positive pre-game mood will show better post-game mood than the participants in a negative pre-game mood group after they are exposed to a losing game

Negative Product Trial and Information Processing

Along with a mood state, this study is also interested in how sport consumers react to a losing game when they are in different mood states. People are expected to incorporate different type of information processing in different situation. This phenomenon has been explained with 'dual information processing system' of Chaiken et al (1996). Chaiken and her colleagues suggested that information be processed with either heuristic or systematic information processing system. Heuristic processing is performed by the application of simple decision rules instead of elaborating on all of the incoming information. The simple decision rules can be from a person's past experience or memory, which facilitate his/her processing similar incoming information. In contrast, systematic processing takes more effort to process the information and results in more elaboration. Therefore, any judgment decision based on systematic processing is thought to be more comprehensive and elaborate (Chaiken et al., 1996). The spectators in a better mood are expected to have less concerns and thoughts on negative product trial (i.e., watching a losing game) than the ones in neutral or negative mood because of the selection of heuristic information processing over systematic information system. Empirical evidence can be found in Batra and Stayman (1990). They measured respondents' cognitive elaboration by counting the number of statements generated after they were manipulated to be in two different mood states (i.e., neutral mood and positive mood). The authors found that people in a positive mood generated statistically less number of statements than the people in neutral mood. Thus, it can be expected that the spectators in a positive mood engage in a heuristic information processing and, as a result, produce less comments and thoughts about negative incoming information (i.e., a losing game) than the ones in a negative mood group. Thus, a hypothesis was generated as below.

Hypothesis 2:

Participants in a positive pre-game mood should generate less statements regarding the losing game than the participants in a negative pre-game mood.

In the two hypotheses, the term 'positive mood group' and 'negative mood group' were used in relative sense than absolute meaning. The positive mood group indicates the participants whose mood state is more positive than the participants in a negative mood group. Thus, the participants in negative mood group do not necessarily have negative affect in absolute term. It simply implies that their mood state is less positive than the ones in a positive mood group.

Method

Participants

Data were collected from 73 students (male = 38, female = 35) who were enrolled in two different classes in sport management program at a large Mid-western university in the United States. The average age of the participants was 20.8 (*SD* = 2.64). A student sample for this study was considered to be viable because of a couple of reasons. First, college students represent a large portion of the spectators of college football games. Second, college spectators' reaction to a losing game is not expected to be different from other populations' reaction in an experimental environment.

Covariates

This study incorporated two covariates of team identification and familiarity to football based on close relationships with dependent measures of the study. Madrigal (1995) found that the correlation between team identification and enjoyment was as high as .41. Wann and Schrader (1997) found a similar result in that spectators with higher team identification scored higher on sport spectating enjoyment in a winning game. Due to the known high correlation, team identification was incorporated as a covariate in the study design.

In addition to team identification, familiarity to football was also included as a covariate in the current study. Familiarity to football variable measured how the participants were familiar to the game of football, its rules, and its strategies. Previous research has showed that spectators with higher team identification are more knowledgeable upon sport and team related information than spectators with lower team identification (Wann, Morris-Shirkey,

Peters, and Suggs, 2002). It was conjectured that the spectators with better knowledge about the football should be able to analyze the game more thoroughly. Thus, in case of a losing game, spectators with good knowledge of football will be aware of the poor strategies in the field and errors that players make, which ignorant spectators would not be able to recognize. The level of knowledge should have positive correlation with the quantity of negative information that spectators process in a losing game because spectators with increased knowledge should be able to identify more negative things in a losing game. Based on the positive relationships of team identification and familiarity to football with spectators game experience, both variables were included as covariates in this study.

Measurements

Three items of Team Identification Index (Trail and James, 2001) were included in the questionnaire to measure the level of psychological attachment to school football team: I consider myself to be a "real" fan of the team; I would experience a loss if I had to stop being a fan of the team; and Being a fan of the team is very important to me. The scale has shown a good validity and internal consistency in previous studies (Fink, Trail, and Anderson, 2002; Trail et al., 2003; Trail and James, 2001). All the items were anchored with seven point Likert scale (1 = strongly disagree, 7 = strongly agree).

Three items were developed for this study to measure how participants were familiar to football. The items asked how familiar they were to football, whether they know the strategies used in football, and whether they actually watch football games. Three items were also anchored with seven point Likert scale (1 = strongly disagree, 7 = strongly agree).

Participants' mood was assessed using four items. The items asked whether they were happy, elated, pleased and in good mood. These items were the most common mood items used in previous studies (i.e., Barone, Miniard, and Romeo, 2000; Lee and Sternthal, 1999). The four items were also anchored in seven point Likert scale (1 = strongly disagree, and 7 = strongly agree).

Procedure

All the participants were randomly divided into a treatment group ($1 free giveaway) and a control group (no free gift) by drawing numbers randomly. All the participants were given a number before the drawing. From a box that has numbers from 1 to 73, the researcher drew 33 numbers to give away an envelop that included one dollar bill. The drawing method was used to make sure that the participants were chosen randomly into two different groups and the experimental situation was very close to real situation (i.e., sport spectators receiving free stuffs randomly at a sporting game). Free award has been utilized in many mood studies to manipulate participants' mood when pre-test is not feasible and it has been proven to be successful (i.e., Isen and Levin, 1972; Blevins and Murphy, 1974). This study did not incorporate any mood measure after the participants received $1 bill. That is based on two reasons. First, previous literature incorporated free cookies, dime, 20 cents worth free gift, etc. to put people in a better mood than their counterparts and it was very successful. For example, Isen, Clark, and Schwarts (1976) used a free stationary that was 20 cents worth. If we assume that there has been 3% inflation annually in average. It would be around 50 cents in current value. The study gave away $1 to the participants in a treatment group and it was highly expected that their mood became better than the ones in a control group. The drawing process should have moved the mood of control group further to a negative side because the treatment group received the $1 bill in the presence of control group, who did not get anything. This method should have maximized the gap between the treatment group and control group. The second, the researcher was worried about the participants' answering two similar scales (i.e., pre and post mood scales) in seven minutes. It has been known as a threat to internal validity and external validity of a research (Hyllegard, Mood, and Morrow, 1996). The participants may be sensitized to the scale and it may influence the participants' answers to the second administration of mood scale. This might be leading to another threat to external validity (i. e., Hawthorne effect) when the participants recognized that they were tested on mood based on the result of a sporting game that they just watched.

All participants (a control group and a treatment group) were asked to fill out the Fan Identification Index (Trail and James, 2001) and familiarity to football items before they were exposed to a video clip containing a losing game of the university football team in 1989. This game was chosen because the participants were not likely to remember or have watched the game. The video clip was an edited version of the game lasting seven minutes, in which all the good plays of the opponent team were purposely shown. Even though Isen, Clark and Schwarts (1976) found the effect of positive mood to be around 20 minutes, the length of the video clip was shorter than that. This is because the participants, in the current study, were exposed to negative information for seven minutes whereas the respondents in Isen et al. were kept in their daily routine. It was a very close game in which the home team lost by one point. The opponent has known to have a better football program than the home team. There was no clear rivalry between the two teams.

After the participants finished watching the video clip, they were asked to fill out four-item mood scale. After answering the four mood items, they were asked to write down what they felt about the game for 10 minutes. In the questionnaire, 13 blank lines were provided for the verbal responses. The researcher told the respondents to ask for extra blank paper if they needed it for additional comments. No respondent did so. The participants generated total of 571 statements regarding the team, players, coach, and the plays in the game. The research simply counted the number of statements and coded for further statistical analyses.

Results

The data were analyzed with a MANCOVA with two covariates of team identification and familiarity to football. In the analysis, the independent variable of mood had two levels (positive and negative) and dependent variables were post-game mood and total number of statements.

The composite mean score of team identification was over the median value of 4 (M = 4.71, SD = 1.93). The level of familiarity to football had composite mean score of 5.04 (SD =

.92) on a seven point scale. The minimum value was 3.33, which indicated that most of the participants were very familiar with football. With the composite mean scores of three constructs (team identification, familiarity to football, and mood), Pearson correlation coefficients were calculated (see Table 1) to see if the covariates met the criterion to be an effective covariate. Hair, Anderson, Tatham, and Black (1998) indicate that an effective covariate should have good correlation with dependent measures. The Pearson correlation between FF (familiarity to football) and post-game mood was -.47 ($p < .001$). The Pearson correlation between TID (team identification) and post-game mood was -.37 ($p < .001$). Thus, the two covariates included in this study met the criterion of Hair et al. (1998). To examine the equivalence of covariance matrices across the groups, Box's test of equality was performed. The results indicated that the two groups' covariance matrices were statistically not different ($p = .133$).

A MANCOVA with two covariates (FF and TID) was performed with the dependent variable of post-game mood and total number of statements. The results indicated that dependent measures were statistically different by groups (Wilks' Lambda = .357, $F = 61.34$, $p < .001$, $\eta_p^2 = .643$). The analysis maintained good level of power (1.0). Follow up univariate analyses indicated that the treatment group showed better post-game mood than the control group ($F = 30.51$, $p < .001$, $\eta_p^2 = .307$) and provided less statements regarding the home team and the game ($F = 98.25$, $p < .001$, $\eta_p^2 = .587$). The results of the MANCOVA supported the first and second hypothesis.

Table 1. Correlations among Dependent Measures (Study 1)

	1	2	3
Total Number of Statements		.343**	.508**
Number of Strong Counterarguments			.060
Number of Moderate Counterarguments			

** Correlation is significant at the .01 level.

Discussion

The first hypothesis was supported. The participants who received $1 before they were exposed to a losing game showed better mood than the participants in the control group. The partial eta square indicated that pre-game mood manipulation explained 30.7% of the post-game mood. Given the small amount of effect size found in two covariates (.044 for familiarity to football and .001 for team identification), the effect of pre-game mood found to be the most significant factor in this analysis. Along with the first hypothesis, the second hypothesis was also supported by the result of the MANCOVA analysis. The control group had more statements regarding the game and the home team than the treatment group, which supported that the participants in negative mood group utilized more systematic information processing than the participants in positive mood group.

Even though study 1 revealed the effect of pre-game mood on post-game mood and cognitive elaboration with good effect size, the study needed to address several limitations before the results could be utilized in more sophisticated manner and with more validity.. The first set of limitations was from its selection of participants. As shown in the studies with student samples, this study also had high level of team identification. Even though the data distribution for TID was quite normal (Skewness: -.50; Kurtosis: -1.16), the lowest value of the composite mean score of TID was 2.67 out of 7 whereas the highest mean score was 7.00. Because of the absence of such cases, data analysis with low end of TID was not feasible. Second, the mean score for FF (familiarity to football) was exceptionally high (M = 5.04). This was also stemmed from the characteristic of the participants. The participants were students majoring sport management. Thus, it can be assumed that they had higher level of interest in sport than other populations on campus.

Another limitation can be found in the nature of the covariates. The covariates of team identification and familiarity to football were included based on the zero-order correlations with dependent variable. However, the correlations by two levels of independent groups (i.e., treatment group and control group) showed different results. Their part correlations with dependant variable of mood was not significant (r = .10 and -.30 for team identification and familiarity to football respectively). Their correlations to total numbers of statements were not significant either (r = -.11 and .18 for team identification and familiarity to football respectively). Hair et al. (1998) indicated that researchers can eliminate the covariate if there is not any substantial improvement with the covariate. Another MANOVA with mood and total number of statements was performed to examine the quality of the covariates based on Hair et al.'s (1998) suggestion. The comparison between MANOVA and MANCOVA results indicated that the covariates actually increased the within-group variance and resulted in decreasing the F statistics from 73.48 to 61.34. In addition to F statistics, the covariates reduced the partial eta square from .677 to .643. Thus, the covariates in this study were found not to improve the results and could be eliminated from the data analyses based on Hair et al. (1998). Based on the results and limitations of the study 1, study 2 was planned using additional theoretical support from affect infusion model (AIM, Forgas, 1995) and elaboration likelihood model (ELM, Petty and Cacioppo, 1986).

Study 2

Study 1 examined whether a manipulated mood before a negative product trial (i.e., a losing home game) influenced consumers' post-consumption mood and cognitive elaboration. To advance the results of the first study, study 2 incorporated a level of personal relevance to a product in research hypotheses. A previous literature called for a study regarding the effect of the strength of prior preference to a product on the resultant attitude from a negative product trial (Jain and Maheswaran, 2000). Jain and Maheswaran (2000) found that preference-inconsistent information was processed more systematically and was counterargued more than preference-consistent information. The preference-inconsistent information is such information that is incongruent to previously held idea about a product. The authors, however, were not able to examine the effect of the strength of prior preference because they manipulated the prior preference to be high for their study. In addition to Jain and Maheswaran (2000), Batra and Stephens (1994) found that mood and emotions evoked by advertisements appeared to influence brand attitude more in low personal relevance (motivation) situations than under high relevance (motivation) situations. However, they could not examine a main effect of mood because the participants' mood was set positive across experimental groups. The current study attempted to test what were not tested in Jain and Maheswaran (2000) and Batra and Stephens (1994) because of their research design.

Study 2 has its theoretical bases on affect infusion model (AIM) of Forgas (1995), dual information processing (Chaiken et al., 1996), and elaboration likelihood model (ELM) of Petty and Cacioppo (1986). Study 2 was designed to identify the characteristics of sport consumers (i.e., in terms of the level of team identification) who are more affectively influenced by a negative game outcome and susceptible to mood manipulation. If those consumers are identified, sport marketers can target those spectators and provide any incentives to make them feel less negatively about the game outcome. When resource is limited, this strategy should be able to make the most use out the limited marketing resources.

Influence of the Mood in Different Levels of Personal Relevance

Previous literature has indicated that the effect of mood should not be the same in different level of personal relevance. As noted earlier, Batra and Stephens (1994) found that mood and emotions evoked by advertisements appeared to influence brand attitude more in low personal relevance situations than under high relevance situation. Theoretical basis can be found in affect infusion model of Forgas (1995). Forgas suggested that the role of mood should be limited when people were performing a task through a preexisting goal, which was termed 'motivated processing' in his affect infusion model. Thus, it can be conjectured that people should be influenced more by mood when they are involved in an event that has less personal relevance. In spectating sport, the level of personal involvement and relevance has been termed as 'team identification'. If the thesis of Forgas can be applied to sport spectating environment, the spectators with low team identification are expected to be influenced more by mood manipulation than the ones with high team identification. This speculation is now linked to the results of the first study, in which a manipulated pre-game mood actually influenced participants' post-game mood. If pre-game mood manipulation works differently for the high team identification group and low team identification group, an interaction between pre-game mood and fan identification is expected. This is the major objective of the current study and a hypothesis was developed based on this theorizing.

Hypothesis 1:

Participants in a positive pre-game mood group will show a better mood after watching a losing game than the participants in a negative pre-game mood and this mood effect will be stronger for participants who are low in team identification.

Cognitive Elaboration by Different Mood State and Personal Relevance

Study 1 measured the total number of statements after a negative product trial to examine consumers' post-product trial mood and information processing. The number of statements generated by participants differed by their mood states as hypothesized. In addition to dual information processing and affect infusion model, elaboration likelihood model (ELM, Petty and Cacioppo, 1986) can be added to explain how people process incoming information based on personal relevance of the information. Petty and Cacioppo (1986) indicated that people processing incoming information and thus persuaded through two different routes; central route and peripheral route. People can use central route when the information has a certain level of personal relevance and when an individual has a capacity of processing the information. This central route involves high elaboration such as evaluation, recall, critical judgment and inferential judgment. On the other hand, people use peripheral route when the information has little personal relevance and they are not capable of processing information, which involves less cognitive elaboration. Combining dual information processing theory (i. e., different information processing by different mood states) and ELM (i. e., different cognitive elaboration by different level of personal relevance), it can be conjectured that cognitive elaboration should be moderated by different mood states of an individual and this effect is expected to be larger in low personal relevance situation. Thus, a group of spectators in a positive mood should be engaged in a less cognitive elaboration (c.f., dual information processing) and, among those, a sub-group with low relevance (i.e., participants with low team identification) should use peripheral route, which results in even less cognitive elaboration. A hypothesis was developed as below.

Hypothesis 2:

Participants in a positive pre-game mood group will show less cognitive elaboration after watching a losing game than the participants in a negative pre-game mood group and this mood effect will be stronger for participants who are low in team identification.

The proposed two hypotheses were tested using a MANOVA. Differently from Study 1, Study 2 did not incorporate any covariate based on the discussion of study1. Instead, personal relevance, measured with team identification, was incorporated as an additional independent variable.

Method

The manipulation and the measurements for study 2 were very similar to Study 1. The data were collected from a larger number of participants than Study 1 and, thus, it was possible to incorporate another independent variable of team identification maintaining proper cell size. In addition to the size of sample, Study 2 solicited data from non-sport related major students to maximize the variance in team identification and to improve the generalizability of the results.

Participants, Material, and Procedures

The data were collected from 127 students (male = 67, female = 62) who were enrolled in the classes in the animal science department and interior design program at a large Midwestern university in the United States. The average age of the participants was 21.03 (*SD* = 3.35). All participants were randomly divided into a treatment group (positive mood, *n* = 60) and a control group (negative mood group, *n* = 69) by drawing. The procedures of the experiment were exactly the same as Study 1. All the participants were asked to fill out a Fan Identification Index (Trail and James, 2001) before they were exposed to the video clip. A manipulation check for mood was not incorporated with the same ground as in the study 1.

After the participants finished watching the video clip, they were asked to fill out three-item mood scale. After answering the three mood items, they were given 10 minutes to write down what they felt about the game and the team. The questionnaire contained 13 blank lines for the verbal responses. The researcher told the respondents to ask for extra blank paper, if needed, for additional comments. No respondent did so. Total of 1,243 statements were generated by the participants

Results

The data were analyzed using a MANOVA. The analysis included independent variables of pre-game mood (positive and negative) and team identification (high and low). The dependent variables included post-game mood and cognitive elaboration which is represented by the total number of statements. The descriptive statistics were calculated with SPSS. The composite means and standard deviations by groups (pre-game mood and team identification) are presented in Table 2. The MANOVA results indicated, as hypothesized, an interaction between pre-game mood and team identification (Wilks' Lambda = .898, $F(2, 124) = 7.07$, $p = .001$; $\eta_p^2 = .102$). Follow-up univariate analyses, however, indicated that the interaction was statistically significant only on post-game mood ($F(1, 125) = 12.68$, $p = .001$; $\eta_p^2 = .092$). The difference in post-game mood was larger in a low team identification group than a high team identification group. In both analyses, power levels were maintained above .92. No interaction was found in the dependent measures of total number of statements $F(1, 125) = 1.70$, $p = .195$; $\eta_p^2 = .013$). Thus, only hypothesis 1 was supported.

Table 2. Descriptive Statistics of Dependent Variables by Groups (Study 2)

	Positive Pre-game Mood		Neutral Pre-game Mood		Total	
	High ID *M(SD)* *N= 31*	LoID *M(SD)* *N = 29*	High ID *M(SD)* *N = 42*	LoID *M(SD)* *N = 27*	High ID *M(SD)* *N = 73*	LoID *M(SD)* *N = 56*
Mood	5.28 (.54)	6.42 (.36)	4.06 (1.17)	4.17 (.77)	4.58 (1.13)	5.34 (1.28)
Total	7.08 (2.04)	6.89 (2.21)	11.61 (1.21)	10.63 (1.50)	10.36 (2.02)	8.70 (2.66)

Along with the hypothesized interaction, main effect of team identification and pre-game mood was also examined. The results indicated that main effects also existed. The group differences were found in terms of pre-game mood (Wilks' Lambda = .317, F $(2, 124)$= 133.61, $p < .001$; $\eta_p^2 = .683$) and team identification (Wilks' Lambda = .757, $F(2, 124)$ = 19.90, $p < .001$; $\eta_p^2 = .243$). Follow up univariate analyses indicated that main effects of pre-game mood were found on the three dependent variables. The post-game mood was found to be statistically different by the pre-game mood ($F(1, 125)$ = 140.26, $p < .001$; $\eta_p^2 = .529$). The participants with better pre-game mood showed better post-game mood. The total number of statements generated also had statistically significant group differences ($F(1, 125)$ = 132.75, $p < .001$; $\eta_p^2 = .515$). The participants in the treatment group showed less number of statements than the ones in the control group.

Discussion

The second study incorporated two independent variables of pre-game mood and personal relevance (i.e., team identification) to examine whether pre-game mood moderate the post-game mood after participants watched a losing game and whether the mood effect was greater in low team identification situation. The results indicated that the participants in the positive pre-game mood showed better post-game mood than the ones in a negative mood group, which replicated the result of study 1 sucessfully. Furthermore, the difference in post-game mood was greater in the low team identification group (see Figure 1) than its counterparts, which supported the argument that mood effect is limited in motivated processing (Forgas, 1995). Thus, we can say that the spectators with low team identification may be more influenced by pre-game mood manipulation than the ones with high team identification.

The participants with better pre-game mood showed that they actually suppressed the cognitive elaboration and generated less statements regarding the game. The mean score for the total number of statements was statistically lower for the participants with positive pre-game mood. The main effect of team identification also followed the pattern. The participants with high identification actually generated more statements regarding the team and the games, which can be explained by their post-game mood. The participants with higher team identification showed worse post-game mood and thus incorporated systematic information system. This result also can be explained with ELM (Petty and Cacioppo, 1986) in that the participants with high level of team identification processed the information with central route that incorporates more cognitive elaboration.

The results partially supported interaction hypotheses. A two-way interaction effect was statistically significant in multivariate analysis. In addition, a follow up univariate analysis supported an interaction hypothesis for post-game mood. This study also hypothesized that two-way interaction should be found in total number of statements. However, the results did not support this. The pre-game mood was found to moderate two dependent measures (i.e., post-game mood and total statements) but its effect was not modified by team identification when dependent measure was the total number of statements.

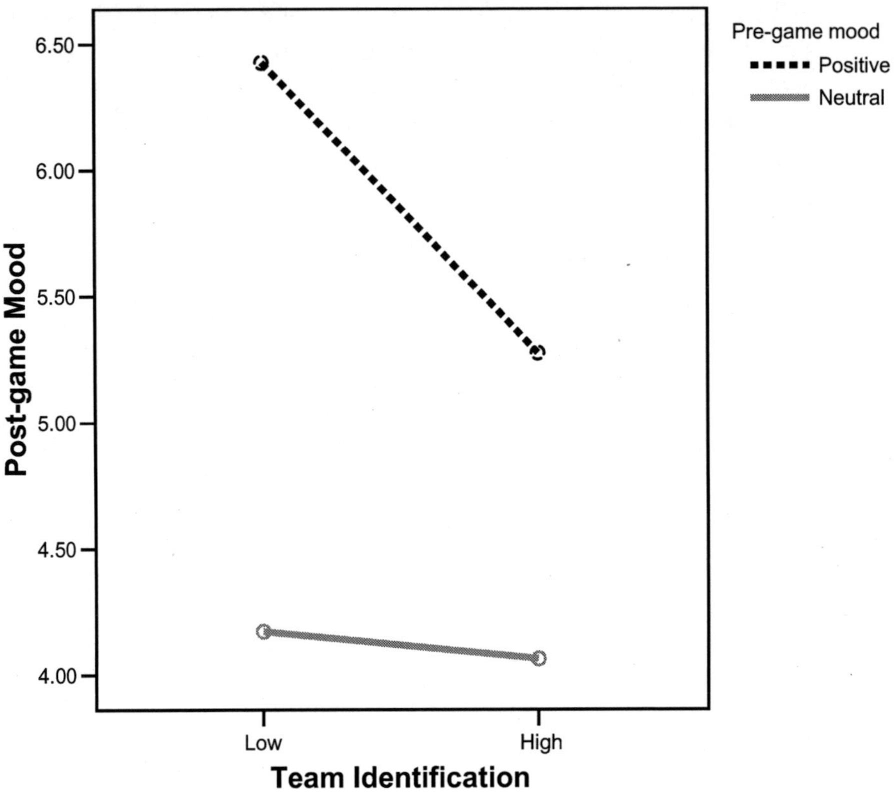

Figure 1. Two-way interaction on post-game mood.

Marketing Implications

The results of the study provide several marketing implications. First, even though there were mixed results in terms of cognitive elaboration, the post-game mood itself was clearly maintained as it was shown in study 1 and 2 as well. The participants in the treatment groups showed better mood than the ones in the control groups in both studies. Second, in addition to the effect of pre-game mood, this study was able to segment a group of people who were more vulnerable to pre-game mood manipulation. The results of the interaction between pre-game mood and team identification found that the participants with low team identification were more influenced by the pre-game mood manipulation than the ones with high team identification. Thus, price oriented promotion or any incentive in a losing game may have the greatest effect on spectators with low team identification. This information is critical to sport marketers when promotional resource is limited. When such resource is limited, for it to be more efficient, sport marketers need to provide money-oriented promotions to customers with low team identification expecting them to have less negative mood after they watched a losing game.

Limitation and Future Research

First limitation came from the length of the video clip used for the studies. The studies revealed, based on the length of the video clip, that the mood of the participants was actually maintained for seven minutes. Not many things can be done seven minutes before a sporting game is over. Thus, to improve practical value of the studies, a future study needs to examine the same effects with longer video clips.

Along with the time length of mood maintenance mechanism, future research also needs to explore possible differences in type of promotion that may manipulate sport spectators mood. This study manipulated the pre-game mood with the free giveaway of $1. However, this kind of promotion is not always feasible for sport organizations. Many different form of mood manipulation (e. g., sample products from outside sponsors, quality of half-time show, etc.) should be tested for the results to be practically applicable to real spectating environment.

Further advancement can be made by improving the generalizability of the study. This study, even though study 2 has more generalizability than study1, is quite limited in terms of generalizability. The study used student sample from one university. This study used American football. Thus, the results of the study cannot be generalized to other populations or different sport settings. Aforementioned shortcomings should be addressed in future research.

References

Alford, J. B., and Sherrell, L. D. (1996). The role of affect in consumer satisfaction judgments of credence based services. *Journal of Business Research, 37*, 71-84.

Barone, M. J., Miniard, P. W., and Romeo, J. B. (2000). The influence of positive mood on brand extension evaluations. *Journal of Consumer Research, 26*, 386-400.

Batra, R., and Stayman, D. M. (1990). The role of mood in advertising effectiveness. *Journal of Consumer Research, 17*, 203-214.

Batra, R., and Stephens, D. (1994). Attitudinal effects of ad-evoked moods and emotions: The moderating role of motivation. *Psychology and Marketing, 11*, 199-215.

Blevins, G., and Murphy, T. (1974). Feeling good and helping: Further phonebooth findings. *Psychological Reports, 34* (Feb), 326.

Bower, G. H. (1981). Mood and memory. *American Psychologist, 36,* 129-148.

Carlson, T. P., and Adams H. E. (1980). Activity valence as a function of mood change. *Journal of Abnormal Psychology, 89*, 368-377.

Chaiken, S., Giner-Sorolla, R., and Chen, S. (1996). Beyond accuracy: Defense and impression motives in heuristic and systematic information processing. In P. M. Gollwitzer and J. A. Bargh (Eds.). *The Psychology of action: Liking motivation and cognition to behavior* (pp. 553-578). New York: Guilford Press.

Clark, M. S., and Isen, A. M. (1982). Toward understanding the relationship between feeling states and social behaviors. In A. Hastorf and A. M. Isen (Eds.), *Cognitive Social Psychology.* New York: Elsevier.

Clark, M. S., and Teasdale, J. D. (1985). Constraints on the effects of mood on memory. *Journal of Personality and Social Psychology, 48*, 1595-1608.

Dube, J., and Menon, K. (2000). Multiple roles of consumption emotions in post-purchase satisfaction with extended service transactions. *International Journal of Service Industry Management, 11*, 287-304.

Fink, J. S., Trail, G. T., and Anderson, D. F. (2002). An examination of team identification: Which motives are most salient to its existence? *International Sports Journal, 6*(Summer), 195-207.

Forgas, J. P. (1995). Mood and judgment: The affect infusion model (AIM). *Psychological Bulletin, 117*(1), 39-66.

Forgas, J. P., Bower, G. H., and Krantz, S. E. (1984). The influence of mood on perceptions of social interactions. *Journal of Experimental Social Psychology, 20*, 497-513.

Hair, J. F., Jr., Anderson, R. E., Tatham, R. L., and Black, W. C. (1998). *Multivariate data analysis* (5th ed.). Upper Saddle River, NJ: Prentice Hall.

Handely, I. M., Lassiter, D. G., Nickell, E. F., and Herchenroeder, L. M. (2004). Affect and automatic mood maintenance. *Journal of Experimental Social Psychology, 20*, 106-112.

Hyllegard, R., Mood, D. P., and Morrow, J. R. (1996). Interpreting research in sport and exercise science. St. Louis, Missouri: Mosby-Year Book Inc.

Isen, A. M. and Levin, P. (1972). Effect of feeling good on helping: Cookies and kindness. *Journal of Personality and Social Psychology, 21,* 384-388.

Isen, A. M., Clark, M., and Schwartz, M. F. (1976). Duration of the effect of good mood on helping: "Footprints on the sands of time." *Journal of Personality and Social Psychology, 34*, 385-393.

Isen, A. M., and Patrick, R. (1983). The effect of positive feelings on risk taking: When the chips are down. *Organizational Behavior and Human Decision Processes, 31,* 194-202.

Isen, A. M., and Simmonds, S. (1978). The effect of feeling good on a helping task that is incompatible with good mood. *Social Psychology Quarterly, 41*, 345-349.

Isen, A. M., Shalker, T. E., Clark, M., and Karp, L. (1978). Affect, accessibility of material in memory, and behavior: A cognitive loop? *Journal of Personality and Social Psychology, 36,* 1-12.

Jain, S. P., and Maheswaran, D. (2000). Motivated reasoning: A depth-of-processing perspective. *Journal of Consumer Research, 26*, 358-371.

Lee, A. Y., and Sternthal, B. (1999). The effects of positive mood on memory. *Journal of Consumer Research, 26,* 115-127.

Lijander, V., and Strandvik, T. (1997). Emotions in service satisfaction. *International Journal of Service Industry Management, 8*, 148-169.

Madrigal, R. (1995). Cognitive and affective determinants of fan satisfaction with sporting event attendance. *Journal of Leisure Research, 27,* 205-227.

Oliver, R. L. (1997). *Satisfaction: A behavioral perspective on the consumer.* New York: McGraw-Hill.

Petty, R. E., and Cacioppo, J. T. (1986). *The elaboration likelihood model of persuasion.* New York: Academic Press.

Trail, G. T., and James, J. D. (2001). The Motivation Scale for Sport Consumption: Assessment of the Scale's Psychometric Properties. *Journal of Sport Behavior, 24,* 108-127.

Trail, G. T., Fink, J. S., and Anderson, D. F. (2003). Sport spectator consumption behavior. *Sport Marketing Quarterly, 12*, 8-17.

Wann, D. L., and Schrader, M. P. (1997). Team identification and the enjoyment of watching a sporting event. *Perceptual and Motor Skills, 84*, 954.

Wann, D. L., Morris-Shirkey, P. A., Peters, E. J., and Suggs, W. L. (2002). Highly identified sport fans and their conflict between expression of sport knowledge and biased assessment of team performance. *International Sports Journal, 6*, 153-159

In: Hot Topics in Sports and Athletics
Editor: Samuel R. Bakere, pp. 79-86
ISBN 978-1-60456-077-0

Chapter 5

Federally Mandated Random Drug Testing in Professional Athletics: Constitutional Issues*

Charles V. Dale

Abstract

Problems of usage of steroids and other performance enhancing drugs in professional and amateur athletics have been the focus of a series of investigative hearings before the House Government Reform Committee. The Committee began taking evidence on March 17, 2005, when several former and current players, medical experts, and major league baseball executives were summoned to testify in the first hearing. Committee Chairman Tom Davis has urged all sports leagues to "acknowledge that their testing programs need improvement" and has framed bipartisan legislation to establish a uniform testing policy for major professional sports leagues. Currently, there are four professional athletic drug testing bills before Congress: S. 1114 (Senator McCain); H.R. 2565 (Representative Davis); H.R. 1862 (Representative Stearns); and H.R. 2516 (Representative Sweeney). The McCain and Davis bills are virtually identical, and all four bills would establish minimum drug standards – including random testing – for some professional sports leagues.

Congressionally mandated drug-testing requirements for both public employees and workers in private industry subject to federal regulation have a fairly long and well established legal history. Nonetheless, the federal courts have recognized limits, largely anchored in constitutional privacy interests of affected workers, that circumscribe governmental authority to impose suspicionless random testing requirements in the public or private sectors. These decisions establish that "compelling" governmental interests may, in appropriate circumstances, override constitutional objections to testing procedures by employees whose privacy expectations are diminished by the nature of their duties or workplace scrutiny to which they are otherwise subject. They further

* Excerpted from CRS Report RL32911, dated June 27, 2005.

suggest, however, that substantial constitutional difficulties probably confront any broad-based testing program that is not limited to specific occupational categories or to persons for whom the government is able to demonstrate some special need to test.

It could be argued that professional players have a diminished expectation of privacy as the consequence of league or association rules that already require routine physical examinations and testing for drugs in certain circumstances. Moreover, a separate argument could be made that safety and health concerns associated with steroid usage, and the importance of professional athletes as role models for the nation's youth, justify unannounced testing for anabolic steroids or other controlled substances. Testing of randomly selected athletes may also be the least intrusive route to an effective steroid detection program. Past major league baseball procedures, it has been argued, do not deter steroid use. Moreover, arguably, the reasonable suspicion standard may be unworkable since most often there may be no outward symptoms to signal the use of steroids.

Problems of usage of steroids and other performance enhancing drugs in professional and amateur athletics have been the focus of a series of investigative hearings before the House Government Reform Committee. The Committee began taking evidence on March 17, 2005, when several former and current players, medical experts, and major league baseball executives were summoned to testify in the first hearing. National Football League Commissioner Paul Tagliabue next testified, on April 27th, concerning details of the NFL steroid testing procedures and how they were negotiated between the league and the NFL players' union. The Committee also requested summaries of all test results during the period that testing has been in place, although not the names of individual players. Similar requests have reportedly been made of National Basketball Association, National Hockey League, US Soccer Federation, Major League Soccer, Association of Tennis Professionals, USA Track and Field, and USA Cycling. Committee Chairman Tom Davis has urged all sports leagues to "acknowledge that their testing programs need improvement" and has framed bi-partisan legislation to establish a uniform testing policy for major professional sports leagues.[1] Currently, there are four professional athletic drug testing bills before Congress: S. 1114 (Senator McCain); H.R. 2565 (Representative Davis); H.R. 1862 (Representative Stearns); and H.R. 2516 (Representative Sweeney). The McCain and Davis bills are virtually identical, and all four bills would establish minimum drug standards – including random testing – for some professional sports leagues.

The McCain/Davis proposal, for example, would require "major professional sports leagues" – defined to include Major League Baseball, the National Football League, the National Basketball Association, and the National Hockey League, and any "successor leagues" – to implement independently administered drug testing programs mirroring the standard of the United States Anti-Doping Agency (USADA). At a minimum, each professional athlete would have to be tested without advance notice no less than five times each calendar year, including at least two offseason tests. Each test would have to cover all substances prohibited in USADA's anti-doping code and would have to be analyzed at a USADA-approved lab.

Athletes testing positive (or refusing to test) a first time must be suspended a minimum of two years and would be subject to permanent suspension from the professional sports association for any later infraction. The leagues would be required to disclose positive tests and resulting penalties to the public. Each covered league would have to develop an adjudication process to provide the athlete who tests positive a hearing (after notice), representation of counsel, and the right to appeal. While such proceedings are pending, the athlete in question would be suspended. For a detailed discussion of all measures currently before Congress on the subject, see CRS Report RS22156, *Drug Testing in Sports: Proposed Legislation*, by Nathan Brooks.

Congressionally mandated drug testing requirements for both public employees and workers in private industry subject to federal regulation have a fairly long and well-established legal history. Nonetheless, as described more fully below, the federal courts have recognized limits, largely anchored in constitutional privacy interests of affected workers, that circumscribe governmental authority to impose suspicionless random testing requirements in the public or private sectors. This report examines relevant judicial precedents for their applicability to the issue of random testing for performance-enhancing substances in professional athletics.

Constitutional Background

Constitutional law on the subject of governmentally mandated drug-testing is primarily an outgrowth of the Fourth Amendment prohibition on unreasonable searches and seizures.[2] A judicial exception to traditional requirements of a warrant and individualized suspicion for "administrative" searches has been applied to random drug testing of government employees, and of private employees tested pursuant to government regulation. In the employment setting, such testing has been justified under a "special needs" analysis, which the courts have applied in relatively narrow circumstances directly implicating "compelling" public safety, law enforcement, or national security interests of the government. More generalized governmental concerns for the "integrity" or efficient operation of the public workplace have usually not been deemed sufficient to justify interference with the "reasonable expectation of privacy" of workers or other individuals to be tested

The Supreme Court in 1989 applied the "special needs" doctrine to dispense with the normal warrant and probable cause requirements of the Fourth Amendment when the government demonstrates compelling justification "beyond ordinary law enforcement" for an employee drug testing program. In *National Treasury Employees Union v. Von Raab*,[3] extraordinary safety and national security concerns justified urinalysis testing of Customs Service employees seeking transfer or promotion to positions directly linked to drug interdiction, handling classified information, or the carriage of firearms. Similarly, in *Skinner v. Railway Labor Executives' Ass'n*,[4] neither a warrant nor particularized suspicion was required for a Federal Railway Administration (FRA) program of blood and urine tests for railroad employees involved in accidents or who violated certain safety standards. In both cases, the Court emphasized that special needs analysis applied only where testing was not used as a prosecutorial tool. In *Veronia School District v. Acton,*[5] the Supreme Court first approved of random drug testing procedures – for high school student athletes rather than public employees – a holding that it later extended to permit random drug testing of students participating in non-athletic extracurricular activities as well. However, the Court distinguished earlier rulings when, in *Chandler v. Miller*,[6] it voided a Georgia law requiring drug testing of candidates for state office because no "special need" substantial enough to warrant suspicionless searches was shown.

The Supreme Court in *Skinner* discarded the reasonable suspicion standard for testing within industries that are "pervasively regulated." The rationale is that the existence of extensive federal or state regulation in and of itself diminishes the reasonable expectation of privacy of those involved in the industry. The primary issue before the lower courts in *Shoemaker v. Handel*[7] was whether state-mandated drug and alcohol tests, administered without individualized suspicion, to thoroughbred race horse jockeys by the New Jersey Racing Commission, violated the Fourth Amendment.

The district court upheld the program, finding that the jockeys voluntarily participated in horse racing and that the state had shown a compelling need for conducting the tests. First, the court recognized that horse racing was a unique class of industry subject to "heavy" state regulation. Second, jockeys were licensed by the state and had received notice of the implementation of the tests. Although notice and licensure did not serve as a waiver of Fourth Amendment rights, they were factors to be considered in balancing the jockey's expectations of privacy against the needs of the state. Third, the state had a vital interest in ensuring that the horse racing industry was run honestly and safely and that the public perceived it as such. Finally, the jockeys tested were selected by random drawing not subject to the bias or discretion of test administrators.

The Third Circuit Court of Appeals affirmed the district court decision. In particular, the appellate opinion emphasized the pervasiveness of New Jersey state regulation and the state's "strong" interest in preserving the "integrity" of the horse-racing industry. In assessing the reasonableness of the testing scheme, the *Shoemaker* court found that the integrity of a sport, from which large sums of revenue were collected, outweighed the jockeys' individual privacy interests.

> New Jersey has a strong interest in assuring the public of the integrity of persons engaged in the horse racing industry. Public confidence forms the foundation for the success of an industry based on wagering. Frequent alcohol and drug testing is an effective means of demonstrating that persons in the horse racing industry are not subject to certain outside influences. It is the public's perception, not the known suspicion, that triggers the state's strong interest in conducting warrantless testing.[8]

Summing up, the Third Circuit concluded that to justify governmentally imposed random testing, there must be a "strong state interest" in the search and "the pervasive regulation of the industry must have reduced the justifiable privacy expectation of the subject of the search."[9] Other post-*Shoemaker* rulings are in agreement.[10]

In *Veronia School District v. Acton,* [11] the Supreme Court sustained a random drug-testing program for high school students engaged in interscholastic athletic competition. The Student Athlete Drug Policy required mandatory and random suspicionless urinalysis testing of all student athletes within the district. The purpose of the policy was to protect the health and safety of the athletes and to rehabilitate drug users by enrolling them in a drug assistance program. All students wanting to participate in a school-sponsored sports team had to provide a consent form, signed both by the student and his or her parents, acquiescing in the tests. Each athlete was tested at the beginning of the athletic season, and anytime during the season that such student's name was randomly selected. Ten percent of the athletes were randomly drawn each week from a pool for testing.

The Supreme Court found that the privacy interest of high school student athletes is diminished by "an element of 'communal undress' inherent in athletic competition." "School sports are not for the bashful," and by choosing to participate in athletics the students "voluntarily subject themselves to a degree of regulation even higher than that imposed on students generally."[12] Moreover, an "immediate crisis," caused by "a sharp increase in drug use" in the school district, triggered installation of the program. District Court findings established that student athletes were not only "among the drug users," they were "leaders of the drug culture."[13] The opinion emphasized that "students within the school environment have a lesser expectation of privacy than members of the public generally."[14]

Balanced against this diminished expectation, the Court determined that the state's interest in protecting the physical and mental well-being of student athletes while in state custody was "important – indeed perhaps compelling." In this regard, the program's context was "central" to Justice Scalia's majority opinion. Local government bears large "responsibilities, under a public school system, as guardian and tutor of children entrusted to its care."[15] Because of this "custodial and tutelary" relationship between the government and its students, school officials regularly exercise "a degree of supervisory control that could not be exercised over free adults."

In *Board of Education v. Earls*,[16] the Court pressed the *Veronia School District* rationale one step further, finding that because of its unique relationship with students, the state's interest in preventing drug use outweighs the privacy interest of students participating in any competitive extracurricular activities. In addition, *Earls* noted "this Court has not required a particularized or pervasive drug problem before allowing the government to conduct suspicionless drug testing"[17] and would not set a threshold level of drug abuse sufficient to support a drug testing program. Instead, the Court found that prevention of harm to school children tested sufficed to demonstrate the necessity for a drug testing policy.

Performance Enhancing Drugs in Professional Sports

These decisions establish that "compelling" governmental interests may, in appropriate circumstances, override constitutional objections to testing procedures by employees whose privacy expectations are diminished by the nature of their duties or workplace scrutiny to which they are otherwise subject. They further suggest, however, that substantial constitutional difficulties probably confront any broadbased testing program that is not limited to specific occupational categories or to persons for whom the government is able to demonstrate some special need to test. A special need has generally been found where there is a history of drug abuse in an industry, when the employment involves work in safety-sensitive or high risk positions, or where there is evidence that drug use has led to accidents or other dangers to the public welfare. But, as Justice Scalia suggests in *Veronia School*

District, the concept may be sufficiently elastic to encompass any "interest that appears *important enough* to justify the particular search at hand, in light of other factors that show the search to be relatively intrusive upon a genuine expectation of privacy."[18] As such, the legality of any mandatory testing regime may depend upon the range of governmental interests that the Court ultimately declares to be "compelling" for Fourth Amendment purposes, and how close the required "nexus" to such interests must be to justify random testing of specific individuals or groups.

The application of the *Shoemaker* precedent would seem to require judicial recognition that professional sports, like horse racing involved there, is a "closely regulated industry." While professional baseball, football, and hockey may be subject to union collective bargaining agreements and other largely self-imposed owners' association and league rules, the hand of government in day- to-day team governance and control appears to be far less. Instead, owners individually and in association remain largely free to set their own standards for player conduct and team management, and even enjoy some limited exemptions from federal regulation – antitrust, for example – that apply to other business sectors. Nor, unlike the jockeys in *Shoemaker*, are professional baseball or football players licensed by state or federal authorities, a potentially relevant distinction. In short, the position of the professional athlete may be readily distinguishable from the jockeys in *Shoemaker* and railroad workers in *Skinner.* For similar reasons, the "custodial and tutelary" relationship of the state to student athletes would appear to deprive *Veronia School District* and its progeny of direct precedential (though perhaps not persuasive) value.

Even apart from governmental regulation, however, it could be countered that professional players have a diminished expectation of privacy as the consequence of league or association rules that already require routine physical examinations and testing for drugs in certain circumstances. Moreover, a separate argument could be made that safety and health concerns associated with steroid usage, and the importance of professional athletes as role models for the nation's youth, justify unannounced testing for anabolic steroids or other controlled substances. Medical evidence could be mustered in the course of ongoing congressional hearings of the adverse health effects, not only to the steroid users, but to the safety of other players. Second, it could be argued, protecting the integrity of the game may be particularly important given the demonstrable influence of professional athletes on young players at all levels. The NFL, for example, cites three reasons, including the health of players, for its concern about the use of prohibited substances.

> [They] threaten the fairness and integrity of the athletic competition on the playing field... [T]he League is concerned with the adverse health effects of steroid use. Although research is continuing, steroid use has been linked to a number of physiological, psychological, orthopedic, reproductive, and other serious health problems . . .[T]he use of Prohibited Substances by NFL players sends the wrong message to young people who may be tempted to use them.[19]

Thus, both the NFL and World Anti-Doping Agency have acknowledged that steroid use can undermine the health of athletes and the fairness of athletic competition.

Finally, testing of randomly selected athletes may be the least intrusive route to an effective steroid detection program. "It seems to us self-evident that a drug problem largely fueled by the 'role model' effect of athletes' drug use, and of particular danger to athletes, is effectively addressed by making sure that athletes do not use drugs."[20] Past major league baseball procedures, it appears, do not deter steroid use. Moreover, arguably, the reasonable suspicion standard may be unworkable since most often there may be no outward symptoms to signal the use of steroids. Thus, the suspicionless, administrative search exception might be the only means of effectively deterring athletes from using steroids. In addition, it may avoid possible problems of subjectivity and prejudice that arguably attend the application of "reasonable cause" or other suspicionbased standards.

References

[1] 4/28/05 *Phila. Daily News* 70, 2005 WLNR 6611442.

[2] Drug testing programs have also been challenged under the First, Fifth, and Fourteenth Amendments, based on arguments that the testing procedures or some other aspect of the program violated rights to due process, equal protection, privacy, and freedom of religion. In general, such claims have proven unsuccessful where the testing program included legal safeguards, such as the use of non-discriminatory testing practices, chain of custody procedures, confidentiality, adequate notice, properly certified laboratories, confirmatory tests, and other procedures designed to ensure fairness and to minimize the intrusiveness of the drug testing program. See, e.g. Shoemaker v. Handel, 795 F.2d 1136, 1139-41, 1143 (referring to selective enforcement of urine testing of jockeys as denying them equal protection of the laws); Rushton v. Nebraska Pub. Power District, 844 F.2d 562, 564-66 (8th Cir. 1988)(discussing plaintiffs' contention that the drug testing program violated their First Amendment rights).

[3] 489 U.S. 656 (1989).

[4] 489 U.S. 602 (1989).

[5] 515 U.S. 646 (1995).

[6] 520 U.S. 305 (1997).

[7] 619 F. Supp. 1089 (D.N.J. 1985), aff'd, 795 F.2d 1136 (3d Cir. 1986).

[8] Id. at 1142.

[9] Id.

[10] See e.g. Dimeo v. Griffin, 943 F.2d 679 (7th Cir 1991)(en banc) where the full appeals court upheld a similar rule of the Illinois Racing Board on behalf of jockeys and other horse racing participants required to submit to suspicionless drug testing. In striking a balance between the intrusiveness of the rule and the Board's reasons for it, the court cited the state's substantial interest in promoting the safety of participants as well as protecting financial revenue which it derive from the betting public's interest in a "clean" sport. The opinion also stressed that since jockeys and other participants were subject to frequent medical examinations, they had a diminished expectation of privacy, which was outweighed by the state's interests in this case.

[11] 515 U.S. 646 (1995).

[12] Id. at 650.

[13] Id at 649.

[14] Id. at 657.

[15] Id. at 665.

[16] 536 U.S. 822 (2002)

[17] Id. at 835.

[18] Id. at 661 (emphasis in original).

[19] National Football League, National Football League Policy on Anabolic Steroids and Related Substances, 2003 (as amended May 15, 2003), p. 1. Similarly, one of the purposes of the World Anti-Doping Program and the World Anti-Doping Code is "[t]o protect the Athletes' fundamental right to participate in doping-free sport and thus promote health, fairness, and equality for Athletes worldwide. . ." World Anti-Doping Agency, World Anti- Doping Code, 2003, ava i l abl e online at [ht t p : / /www.wadaama. org/rtecontent/document/code_v3.pdf], p. 1.

[20] Veronia, 515 U.S. at 636.

In: Hot Topics in Sports and Athletics
Editor: Samuel R. Bakere, pp. 87-113

ISBN 978-1-60456-077-0

Chapter 6

Anti-Doping Policies: The Olympics and Selected Professional Sports*

L. Elaine Halchin

Abstract

The use of performance-enhancing substances by athletes has a long history, predating the ancient Greek Olympiads. Concern about this practice was manifested in the 20th century by, in the case of the Olympics, the creation of anti-doping organizations, and the adoption of anti-doping policies by these organizations and professional sports leagues in the United States. Leading the way was the International Olympic Committee (IOC), which implemented testing in 1968 at the Olympic Games in Grenoble, France, and Mexico City, Mexico. The National Basketball Association (NBA) and the National Football League (NFL) followed suit in the 1980s. Major League Baseball implemented an anti-drug policy in 2003.

This report compares current anti-doping policies for performance enhancing substances among the Olympic movement and three professional sports — Major League Baseball, the NBA, and the NFL. Details associated with each of the selected group's policy are presented in Table 1. The report also presents elements of what have been identified as model anti-doping policies and (in the appendix) provides a comparison of Major League Baseball's former and current anti-doping policies (Table 2) and a glossary of related terms.

In general, the report indicates that the anti-doping policies for the Olympic movement are more independent of the sports they regulate than are the policies of Major League Baseball, the NBA, and the NFL, both in the manner in which they are established and in the entities responsible for their implementation. For example, the World Anti-Doping Agency (WADA) unilaterally established the anti-doping policy for Olympic athletes, whereas the professional sports leagues' policies are the result of negotiations with their respective players associations. The Olympic movement also maintains the most comprehensive list of prohibited substances and methods, and provides sanctions that are more strict than in the professional sports. For example, the

* Excerpted from CRS Report RL32894, dated April 29, 2005.

Olympic standard provides a two-year ban for a first violation, whereas Major League Baseball imposes a 10-day suspension without pay for a first violation. Also, Olympic athletes and NFL players are responsible for what is in their bodies, but neither Major League Baseball nor the NBA addresses this subject.

Direct comparison of these sports is sometimes difficult because the policies use different terminology or make reference to other standards. The policies are also constantly changing in response to the development of new substances that are sometimes designed to avoid detection. In some cases, the policies prohibit certain substances for which tests are not available in order to inform athletes about harmful substances. However, in other cases, tests and sanctions are not provided for substances for which tests are available. For example, except for "reasonable cause" testing, Major League Baseball's policy provides for testing and sanctions only with regard to steroids — not other substances prohibited in the league's policy.

This report will be updated as anti-doping policies change and elements of those policies become clearer.

Anti-Doping Policies

While the use of drugs and other substances — such as alcohol, ether, strychnine, anabolic steroids, stimulants, and hallucinogenic mushrooms — as a means of improving athletic performance has a lengthy history, predating the ancient Greek Olympiads, condemnation of the practice did not surface until the early 20th century.[1] In 1933, Dr. Otto Reiser commented that

> [t]he use of artificial means [*to improve performance*] has long been considered wholly incompatible with the spirit of sport and has therefore been condemned. Nevertheless, we all know that this rule is continually being broken, and that sportive competitions are often more a matter of doping than of training. It is highly regrettable that those who are in charge of supervising sport seem to lack the energy for the campaign against this evil, and that a lax, and fateful, attitude is spreading."[2]

Despite such concerns about the use of performance-enhancing substances (PES) by athletes, anti-doping policies for the Olympic movement and major professional sports leagues in the United States were not drafted until the latter part of the 20th century.

- The International Olympic Committee (IOC) implemented testing in 1968, at the Olympic Games in Grenoble, France, and Mexico City, Mexico. Anabolic steroids were added by the IOC to its list of prohibited substances in 1976.[3]
- The National Football League (NFL) followed suit, in 1982, when it began to test players, although testing for anabolic steroids did not begin until 1987.[4] The NFL and the players association have updated their anti-doping policy several times since then. In testimony he presented at a congressional hearing in April 2005, the Commissioner of the NFL stated that the league and the players association recently had agreed to several changes to their policy and that the changes will take effect in 2005.[5] However, because these changes have not been formally published yet, this report treats their last public policy as the current policy.

- The National Basketball Association's (NBA) first anti-doping policy was issued in 1983, and it has been updated several times.[6]
- Major League Baseball implemented an anti-doping policy in 2003. Apparently in response to public pressure, Major League Baseball and the Major League Baseball Players Association (MLBPA) reopened the collective bargaining agreement in 2005 and updated the policy. Although the 2005 policy has not been ratified yet by the players, it appears to be in effect and is treated in this report as the current policy.

This report compares current anti-doping policies among the Olympic movement and three professional sports — Major League Baseball, the NBA, and the NFL.[7] However, this issue clearly transcends these three leagues and the Olympics, and affects other professional sports and amateur athletics. Details associated with each of the selected group's policy are presented in Table 1. Although the antidoping policies in this report sometimes include so-called "recreational" drugs such as cocaine and marijuana, this report generally focuses on performance-enhancing substances. Also, it is important to emphasize that the descriptions and comparisons made here reflect the different sports' anti-doping *policies*, not their *implementation*. In addition, this report presents elements of what have been identified as model antidoping policies and, in the appendix, provides a comparison of Major League Baseball's former and current anti-doping policies (Table 2) and a glossary of related terms.

Olympic Policies More Independent of Regulated Sports

In general, this report indicates that the anti-doping policies for the Olympic movement are more independent of the sports they regulate than are the policies of Major League Baseball, the NBA, and the NFL, both in the manner in which they are established and in the entities responsible for their implementation. For example, the anti-doping policies of the professional sports leagues are established through a collective bargaining process between a players association and the applicable league, both of which benefit from professional players' performances. These policies also are administered by entities selected by the players associations and the leagues (for example, the members of baseball's Health Policy Advisory Committee are selected by Major League Baseball and the Major League Baseball Players Association). By contrast, in the Olympic movement, the World Anti-Doping Agency (WADA) unilaterally established the anti-doping policy and has no vested interested in the athletes' performances. The organization which administers this policy for U.S. Olympic athletes, the U.S. Anti-Doping Agency (USADA), also is independent of athletes and the organization that supports these athletes, the USOC.[8]

Table 1. Comparison of Selected Features of Anti-Doping Policies

	Olympic Movement	**Major League Baseball MLB) and Major League Baseball Players Association (MLBPA) (2005 policy)a**	**National Basketball Association (NBA) and National Basketball Players Association (NBPA)**	**National Football League (NFL) and National Football League Players Association (NFLPA)**
— What organization or individual is responsible for administering the anti-doping policy?	— U.S. Anti-Doping Agency (for American athletes).	— Health Policy Advisory Committee (HPAC).	— Medical director.	— NFL Advisor on Anabolic Steroids and Related Substances.
— Is the organization or individual independent from the sponsoring organization(s)?	— Yes.	— No. MLB and MLBPA each select two members of the HPAC.	— No. The medical director is selected jointly by the NBA and NBPA.	— No. The program is conducted under the auspices of the NFL Management Council, and it appears that the Advisor is an employee of the NFL.b
Is testing conducted offseason (or out of competition, for the Olympics)?	Yes.	Yes.	No, except possibly for "reasonable cause" testing.[c]	Yes.
Is an athlete responsible for prohibited substances found in his or her body?	Yes.	Subject is not addressed in the policy.	Subject is not addressed in the policy.	Yes.
Does the responsible organization test athletes for all prohibited substances?	No.[f]	No (steroids only).[g]	Yes.[f]	No.[f]

Table 1. Comparison of Selected Features of Anti-Doping Policies (Continued)

	Olympic Movement	Major League Baseball MLB) and Major League Baseball Players Association (MLBPA) (2005 policy)a	National Basketball Association (NBA) and National Basketball Players Association (NBPA)	National Football League (NFL) and National Football League Players Association (NFLPA)
Does the anti-doping policy prohibit:[d]				
— Steroids	— Yes.	— Yes.	— Yes.	— Yes.
— Hormones and related substances	— Yes.	— Yes.[h]	— No.	— Yes.[i]
— Beta-2 agonists	— Yes.	— Unclear[j]	— No.	— Yes.
— Agents with antiestrogenic activity	— Yes.	— Unclear.[k]	— No.	— No.
— Diuretics and other masking agents	— Yes.	— Unclear.[l]	— Unclear.[m]	— Yes.
— Enhancement of oxygen transfer	— Yes.	— No.	— No.	— No.
— Chemical and physical manipulation	— Yes.	— Unclear.[l]	— Unclear.m	— Yes.
— Gene doping	— Yes.	— No.	— No.	— No.
— Stimulants	— Yes.	— Unknown, except for ephedra, which is prohibited but not tested.[n]	— Yes, but only amphetamine and its analogues.	— Yes.
— Glucocorticosteroids	— Yes, but only in competition.	— Unclear.[o]	— No.	— No.
— Beta-blockers	— Yes, but only for certain sports.	— Unclear.[p]	— No.	— No.

Table 1. Comparison of Selected Features of Anti-Doping Policies (Continued)

	Olympic Movement	Major League Baseball MLB) and Major League Baseball Players Association (MLBPA) (2005 policy)a	National Basketball Association (NBA) and National Basketball Players Association (NBPA)	National Football League (NFL) and National Football League Players Association (NFLPA)
What laboratory tests the samples?	WADA-accredited laboratories or as otherwise approved by WADA.	Subject is not addressed in the policy, but MLB has indicated that testing is conducted at a WADAaccredited laboratory in Montreal.[q]	Laboratories are selected by the medical director, approved by the NBA and NBPA, and certified by the International Olympic Committee and/or the College of American Pathologists (for steroids), or the Substance Abuse and Mental Health Services Administration (for substances other than steroids).[r]	Under the existing collective bargaining agreement, samples to be analyzed for prohibited substances are to be submitted to the UCLA Olympic Analytical Laboratory at the UCLA School of Medicine.[s]
Are sanctions applicable to all prohibited substances?	Yes.	No (steroids only).[t]	Yes.	Yes.[u]

Table 1. Comparison of Selected Features of Anti-Doping Policies (Continued)

	Olympic Movement	Major League Baseball MLB) and Major League Baseball Players Association (MLBPA) (2005 policy)a	National Basketball Association (NBA) and National Basketball Players Association (NBPA)	National Football League (NFL) and National Football League Players Association (NFLPA)
What are the sanctions for testing positive?				
— First violation	— Two-year ban[v]	— Steroids: 10-day suspension without pay.	— Steroids: Five-game suspension and required to enter steroids program. Amphetamines: First-year player is dismissed from the NBA for one year and required to enter treatment program. A veteran player is dismissed from the NBA for a minimum of two years.[w]	— Suspended without pay for a minimum of four games.
— Second violation	— Lifetime ban.	— 30-day suspension without pay.	— Steroids: 10-game suspension and required to enter steroids program.	— Suspended without pay for a minimum of six games.
— Third violation	— Not applicable.	— 60-day suspension without pay.	— Steroids: 25-game suspension and required to enter steroids program.	— Suspended without pay for at least 12 months.
— Fourth violation	— Not applicable.	— One-year suspension without pay.	— Steroids: Same as third violation.	— Not addressed.
— Subsequent violation(s)	— Not applicable.	— MLB Commissioner imposes further discipline.	— Steroids: Same as third violation.	— Not addressed.

Table 1. Comparison of Selected Features of Anti-Doping Policies (Continued)

	Olympic Movement	Major League Baseball MLB) and Major League Baseball Players Association (MLBPA) (2005 policy)a	National Basketball Association (NBA) and National Basketball Players Association (NBPA)	National Football League (NFL) and National Football League Players Association (NFLPA)
What types of specimens are collected and tested?	Blood or urine.	Urine.	Urine. However, the medical director has authority to determine the use of blood, breath, or other testing techniques.	Urine.

Sources: U.S. Anti-Doping Agency, *United States Anti-Doping Agency Protocol for Olympic Movement Testing*, revised Aug. 13, 2004, available at [http://www.usantidoping.org/files/active/what/protocol.pdf]; U.S. Anti-Doping Agency, "USADA Press Ki t " Jan. 2005, available at [http://www.usantidoping.org/files/active/resources/press_kits/2005%20Fact%20Sheet.pdf]; World Anti-Doping Agency, *World Anti-Doping Code*, 2003, available at [http://www.wada-ama.org/rtecontent/document/code_v3.pdf]; World Anti-Doping Agency, *International Standard for Testing*, June 2003, available at [http://www.wada-ama.org/rtecontent/document/testing_v3_a.pdf]; World Anti-Doping Agency, *International Standard for Therapeutic Use Exemptions*, n.d., available at [http://www.wada-ama.org/rtecontent/document/international_standard.pdf]; World Anti-Doping Agency, *The 2005 Prohibited List, International Standard*, n.d., available at [http://www.wada-ama.org/rtecontent/document/list_book_2005_en.pdf]; Major League Baseball, *Major League Baseball's Joint Drug Prevention and Treatment Program*, n.d., available at [http://reform.house.gov/UploadedFiles/031705%20MLB%20Policy.pdf]; National Basketball Players Association, *NBPA Collective Bargaining Agreement*, n.d., available at [http://www.nbpa.com/cba]; National Football League, *National Football League Policy on Anabolic Steroids and Related Substances*, 2003 (as amended May 15, 2003).

Notes:

a. The policy negotiated by Major League Baseball and the players association that takes effect during the 2005 season has not yet been ratified by the players, but apparently it is in effect. An article issued by *MLB.com* stated that an outfielder for the Tampa Bay Devil Rays tested positive for steroid use and, as a result, was suspended for the10 days. (Barry M. Bloom, "Rays' Sanchez Suspended for 10 Days," *MLB.com*, Apr. 3, 2005, available at [http://mlb.mlb.com/NASApp/mlb/mlb/news/mlbsearcharchive.jsp].

b. The NFL Management Council oversees policies that relate to players, including the collective bargaining agreement. The council reports to the Commissioner of the National Football League. (Information provided by telephone by the NFL Communications Department to the author on Apr. 18, 2005.)

c. Reasonable cause testing is conducted when the Independent Expert who has been selected by the NBA and the NBPA has determined "there is reasonable cause to believe that the player in question has been engaged in the use, possession, or distribution of a Prohibited Substance." (National Basketball Players Association, *NBPA Collective Bargaining Agreement*, n.d., available at [http://www.nbpa.com/cba], Sec. 5(a).)

d. The detail and extent of an anti-doping policy's list of prohibited substances and methods vary from organization to organization. One possible reason for variations among the lists is that some substances may benefit only athletes in certain sports. For example, beta-blockers, which decrease the heart rate and may aid in decreasing tremors or shaking, may be used by athletes who participate in sports that reward precision and accuracy, such as archery.

e. The use of the term "steroids" in this context refers to anabolic or anabolic androgenic steroids, substances which may help an athlete increase his or her muscle size and strength and recover more quickly from injury. The class of substances known as "steroids" includes other types of substances. See "anabolic androgenic steroids" and "steroids" in the glossary.

f. In some cases, accurate laboratory tests do not exist for certain prohibited substances or levels. In other cases, though (e.g., the NFL's policy on human growth hormone), tests are available to detect the prohibited substances but are not used. The NBA tests for all prohibited substances, but its list of such substances is shorter than the lists for the other sports.

g. The federal government has established five schedules of controlled substances. The following three criteria are used to determine on which schedule to place a substance or drug: its potential for abuse, whether the item has a currently accepted medical use in the United States, and the probability that abuse of the substance could lead to physical or psychological dependence. Schedule I includes substances and drugs that have a high potential for abuse, that currently have no accepted medical use in the United States, and that lack accepted safety for use under medical supervision. Substances and drugs listed on one of the remaining four schedules have currently accepted medical uses, and the potential for abuse and the probability that abuse could lead to physical or psychological dependence declines from Schedule II through Schedule IV. (21 U.S.C. § 812(a) and (b).) Major League Baseball's list of prohibited substances includes drugs of abuse (cocaine, LSD, marijuana, opiates, Ecstasy, GHB, PCP, ephedra, all drugs or substances listed on Schedule II, and all Schedule I drugs listed on Addendum B of the league's anti-doping policy) and all anabolic androgenic steroids listed on Schedule III. Section 3.B. of this policy explicitly excludes drugs of abuse from the testing program: "Except as set forth in Section 3.C. [reasonable cause testing], Players shall not be subject to testing for the use of any Drug of Abuse." (Major League Baseball, *Major League Baseball's Joint Drug Prevention and Treatment Program*, n.d., pp. 3 and 6, available at [http://reform.house.gov/UploadedFiles/ 031705%20MLB%20Policy.pdf].)

h. Human growth hormone (hGH) is on the list of prohibited substances, under the heading "steroids," but MLB does not test for it. In testimony offered during a House Committee on Government Reform hearing, Robert D. Manfred Jr., Executive Vice President, MLB, and Elliot J. Pellman, M.D., Medical Advisor to the Commissioner of Baseball, indicated that Major League Baseball does not test for human growth hormone (hGH). The rationale they offered was that no valid urine-based test exists. Mr. Manfred added: "Contrary to published reports, there is not an available, verified test for HGH, even with a blood sample." (U.S. Congress, House Committee on Government Reform, statements of Robert D. Manfred Jr., Executive Vice President, Major League Baseball, and Elliot J. Pellman, M.D., Medical Advisor the Commissioner of Baseball, unpublished hearing, 109th Cong., 1st sess., Mar. 17, 2005, available at [http://mlb.mlb.com/NASApp/mlb/news/press_releases/intro.jsp] and [http://reform.house.gov/Uploaded Files/Pellman%20Testimony.pdf].) It should be noted that the World Anti-Doping Agency tested athletes for hGH at the 2004 Athens Olympics, using a blood test that had been developed and validated in partnership with the IOC and USADA. (World Anti Doping Agency, "Minutes of the WADA Executive Committee Meeting," Nov. 20, 2004, p. 20, available at [http://www.wada-ama. org/en/dynamic.ch2?pageCategory_id=44].)

i. As an example of how the lists of prohibited substances vary from organization to organization, only human growth hormone, animal growth hormone, and human chorionic gonadotropin are included on the NFL's list of hormones. The WADA list includes several other hormones and related substances. (World Anti-Doping Agency, *International Standard for Testing*, June 2003, available at [http://www.wada-ama.org/rtecontent/document/testing_v3_a.pdf].)

j. The list of prohibited substances includes all of Schedule II and an extensive list of substances from Schedule I. It is unclear whether any substances known as "beta-2 agonists" are listed on either of these schedules. Efforts to obtain clarification o n this matter from Major League Baseball or the players association are continuing.

k. The list of prohibited substances includes all of Schedule II and an extensive list of substances from Schedule I. It is unclear whether any substances known as agents with antiestrogenic activity are listed on either of these schedules. Efforts to obtain clarification on this matter from Major League Baseball or the players association are continuing.

l. Masking substances (and methods) are not identified on the list of prohibited substances, but the policy states: "Attempts to substitute, dilute, mask, or adulterate a specimen sample are considered a positive test result." (Major League Baseball, *Major League Baseball's Joint Drug Prevention and Treatment Program*, p. 6.)

m. Masking substances (and methods) are not identified on the list of prohibited substances. However, the policy states that "[if a player attempts to substitute, dilute, mask, or adulterate a specimen sample or in any other manner [alter] a test result," such activity or action will be considered a positive test. (National Basketball Players Association, *NBPA Collective Bargaining Agreement*, Sec. 4(c)(iv).)

n. The list of prohibited substances includes all of Schedule II and an extensive list of substances from Schedule I. It is unclear whether any substances known as stimulants are listed on either of these schedules. Efforts to obtain clarification on this matter from Major League Baseball or the players association are continuing. While ephedra is a prohibited substance, it is found on the "Drugs of Abuse" list, which means it is not included in regular testing of players. (Major League Baseball, *Major League Baseball's Joint Drug Prevention and Treatment Program*, p. 3.)

o. The list of prohibited substances includes all of Schedule II and an extensive list of substances from Schedule I. It is unclear whether any substances known as glucocorticosteroids are listed on either of these schedules. Efforts to obtain clarification on this matter from Major League Baseball or the players association are continuing.

p. The list of prohibited substances includes all of Schedule II and an extensive list of substances from Schedule I. It is unclear whether any substances known as beta-blockers are listed on either of these schedules. Efforts to obtain clarification on this matter from Major League Baseball or the players association are continuing.

q. Major League Baseball and the players association agreed, in spring 2004, to have all drug testing conducted by the Doping Control Laboratory at the INES-Instituted Armand-Flapper Research Center in Montreal. This is a WADA-accredited laboratory. (Major League Baseball, "MLB Drug-Testing Programs Move to Olympic-Certified Laboratories," May 11, 2004, available at [http://mlb.mlb.com/NASApp/mlb/content/printerfriendly/Mb/y2004/m05/d11/c740823.jsp].)

r. The Substance Abuse and Mental Health Services Administration is an agency within the Department of Health and Human Services.

s. This is a WADA-accredited laboratory.

t. This sanction is specific to Articles 2.1 (presence of a prohibited substance in an athlete's substance), 2.2 (use or attempted use of a prohibited substance or a prohibited method), and 2.6 (possession of prohibited substances and methods) in the WADA *Code*. For the list of sanctions imposed for other violations, see the WADA *Code*, pp. 27-35. An athlete who has been banned under the WADA *Code* has been declared ineligible. An athlete's status during eligibility is as follows: "No Person who has been declared ineligible may, during the period of ineligibility, participate in any capacity in a Competition or activity (other than authorized anti-doping education or rehabilitation programs) authorized or organized by a Signatory or Signatory's member organization" (p. 35). Signatories are those organizations that have signed and agreed to comply with the WADA *Code* and include "the International Olympic Committee, International Federations, International Paralympic Committee, National Olympic Committees, National Paralympic Committees, Major Event Organizations, National Anti-Doping Organizations, and WADA." (World Anti-Doping Agency, *World Anti-Doping Code*, 2003, available at [http://www.wada-ama.org/ rtecontent/document/code_ v3.pdf], pp. 35, 75.) For example, the list of organizations that have accepted the WADA *Code* includes the International Fencing Federation, International Swimming Federation, International Tennis Federation, and the International Wrestling Federation. (World Anti-Doping Agency, "List of Sports Organizations Who Have Accepted the Code," n.d., available at [http://www.wada-ama.org/en/print.asp?p=42255].)

u. It is unclear what sanction, if any, the NFL would impose on a player who uses masking agents or otherwise practices pharmacological, chemical or physical manipulation of a sample. Both masking agents and doping methods (that is, manipulation) are included on the list of prohibited substances. However, the policy states that "Any effort to substitute, dilute, or adulterate a specimen or to alter a test result may subject a player to more severe discipline than would have been imposed for a positive test." (National Football League, *National Football League Policy on Anabolic Steroids and Related Substances*, pp. 4, 11-12.) The use of the word "may" suggests that the NFL may exercise discretion when dealing with a player who has attempted to alter, or has altered, a test. The phrase "than would have been imposed for a positive test" suggests that the NFL does not treat test alteration the same as a positive laboratory test for a prohibited substance. Efforts to resolve this matter are ongoing.

v. Apparently, these sanctions apply only to positive tests for steroids. As noted above, testing for other substances and drugs prohibited by the league will not be done as part of its ongoing testing program (though players may be tested for these other substances when reasonable cause exists). Nevertheless, it bears noting that no sanctions are included for positive tests of other substances. The 2005 draft of Mb's anti-doping policy states that, for first through fourth violations, a fine may be levied in lieu of imposing a suspension. (Major League Baseball, *Major League Baseball's Joint Drug Prevention and Treatment Program*, n.d., pp. 11-12.) However, as reported in the *Washington Post* on Mar. 21, 2005, both parties (MB and MLBPA) have agreed to eliminate fines, leaving suspensions as the only sanction. ("Agreement Reached to Drop Fines," *Washington Post*, Mar. 21, 2005, p. D5.)

w. Apparently, the MBA's policy does not mention what, if any, penalties are imposed for subsequent violations involving the use of amphetamines.

A comparison of selected features of anti-doping policies shows, among other things, that the Olympic movement maintains the most comprehensive list of prohibited substances and methods. This may be due, at least in part, to the general understanding that some substances or drugs benefit only athletes in certain sports.[9] For example, a drug that slows down heart rate and reduces fine motor tremors would be more helpful to an archer than a basketball player. Another feature on which the Olympic movement and most professional sports leagues differ is whether an athlete is responsible for the substances discovered is in his or her body. In both the Olympics and the NFL, an athlete is responsible, but neither Major League Baseball nor the NBA addresses this subject in their written policies. Sanctions for testing positive also vary. The Olympic movement imposes the most stringent penalties: the first violation results in a two-year ban, and a second violation results in a lifetime ban from competition, as defined by WADA.[10] In contrast, according to Major League Baseball's current policy, a second violation results only in a 30-day suspension without pay.

Issues in Comparing Anti-Doping Policies

The structure and content of these sports' anti-doping policies vary in a number of ways, including the subjects covered in those policies, the extent of detail provided, and the language and terminology used to identify or describe prohibited substances. As a result, direct comparison of the policies is extremely difficult, and certain of their provisions may be subject to differing interpretations. Also, various contextual factors need to be considered when comparing the different sports' antidoping policies.

Identifying Prohibited Substances/Methods

It is sometimes difficult to determine which specific substances and methods are prohibited in an anti-doping policy. As a result, it is difficult to compare those policies. These difficulties can arise when different policies use different terminology, or when a policy refers to an associated statute or standard. For example, Major League Baseball's list of prohibited substances incorporates, by reference, several of the federal government's lists of controlled substances.[11] Examples of substance names found on one of the lists of controlled substances are clonitazene, etoxeridine, and the bacon. However, it is not clear whether any of these substances are beta-2 agonists, agents with antiestrogenic activity, glucocorticosteroids, or beta-blockers — classes of substances identified by WADA as performance-enhancing substances. Our efforts to obtain clarification from Major League Baseball or the players association on this and other matters are continuing.

Changing Nature of Policies

The nature of the problem of doping in sports has implications for the creation of lists of prohibited substances and testing policies. In some cases, performance enhancing substances being used by athletes may not appear on the lists of prohibited substances because sports officials are not aware of their existence or use. For example, in an effort to evade detection of steroid use, some athletes use designer steroids, which are described as follows:

> ... a designer or "new" steroid [is a substance that] has been chemically produced (synthesized in the laboratory)[and] that retains the anabolic properties desired for such a drug. At the same time the molecular structure ... is chemically altered so that the currently used steroid screening test will not ... [find the drug in an athlete's specimen] ....[12]

When it was created, tetrahydrogestrinone (THG) was a designer steroid. THG became known after a then-anonymous track and field coach in the United States provided a sample to USADA, which forwarded the sample to the UCLA Olympic Analytic Laboratory. Using this sample, the laboratory was able to identify the substance.[13] Because designer steroids are developed specifically to avoid detection, it is impossible for anti-doping organizations or sports leagues to include them on their lists of prohibited substances. Therefore, as new doping methods become known, anti-doping policies must be revisited from time to time to ensure they are up to date.

Some of the professional sports included in this report have recently changed their anti-doping policies. The NFL's April 2005 change reportedly tripled the number of times a player can be tested for steroids during the offseason, added to the league's list of prohibited substances, and allowed for retesting of a players' urine samples for designer steroids that may have been previously undetected.[14] A comparison of Major League Baseball's former and current policies (Table 2 in the appendix) also shows several significant differences. Under the former policy, hormones may not have been prohibited; the list of sanctions allowed first-time offenders to be placed in a treatment program and permitted the imposition of a fine in lieu of a suspension without pay for second through fifth violations; and testing was not conducted during the off-season. The current policy prohibits the use of hormones, imposes a 10-day suspension without pay for a first violation and progressively longer suspensions without pay for subsequent violations, and testing is conducted during the off-season.

No Tests or Sanctions for Some Prohibited Substances

Anti-doping policies may not provide tests or sanctions for certain prohibited substances. In some cases, tests for those substances are available, but are not being used. For example, Section 3.B. of Major League Baseball's policy explicitly states that, except for "reasonable cause" testing, "Players shall not be subject to testing for the use of any Drug of Abuse."[15] Notably, included among the list of "drugs of abuse" is ephedra, which the league banned in the wake of a player's death in 2003. Therefore, although a test for ephedra is available, it is not currently included in the list of substances for which players are being tested. In fact, other than "reasonable cause" testing, Major League Baseball's policy does not provide for testing or sanctions for any prohibited substance other than steroids.[16]

In other cases, though, lists of prohibited substances may include known substances for which there are no laboratory tests, or, in the case of hormones and other substances that occur naturally in the human body, for which there is an insufficient amount of data to determine "what levels of ... hormones are abnormal or indicative of abuse and what levels are normal."[17] For example, natural hormones other than testosterone — such as human chorionic gonadotropin, insulin, and erythropoietin — may be found on lists of prohibited substances, but laboratory tests may not be available yet and what constitutes an abnormal level in the human body may not yet have been determined.

Nevertheless, including substances for which laboratory tests do not exist on a list of prohibited substances may serve an organization's purposes. For example, an organization may establish a list not only to alert athletes to doping tests but also to inform them about harmful substances. One of the purposes of the World Anti- Doping Program and the *World Anti-Doping Code* is "[t]o protect the Athletes' fundamental right to participate in doping-free sport and thus promote health, fairness and equality for Athletes worldwide ...."[18] Certain elements of the rationale for the *Code* may also have a bearing on the inclusion of substances for which tests are not yet available. These include, for example, "ethics, fair play and honesty .... health .... character and education .... respect for rules and laws .... respect for self and other participants ...."[19] The National Football League cites three reasons, including the health of players, for its concern about the use of prohibited substances:

> [They] threaten the fairness and integrity of the athletic competition on the playing field .... [T]he League is concerned with the adverse health effects of steroid use. Although research is continuing, steroid use has been linked to a number of physiological, psychological, orthopedic, reproductive, and other serious health problems .... [T]he use of Prohibited Substances by NFL players sends the wrong message to young people who may be tempted to use them.[20]

Thus, it appears that these two organizations (WADA and the NFL), and possibly others as well, recognize that the value of an anti-doping program or policy extends beyond testing to include messages about harmful substances and how they might undermine other aspects of athletic competition.

Comparison of Olympic Movement, Major League Baseball, NBA, and NFL Anti-Doping Policies

Table 1 below compares specific elements of the anti-doping policies of the Olympic movement, Major League Baseball, the NBA, and the NFL. Those elements include which organizations administer the policies, the substances and methods prohibited, and the sanctions for testing positive for a prohibited substance. In many cases, reference to an associated footnote is needed to understand particular elements of a sport's policy.

Elements of Model Anti-Doping Policies

Experts in the field of drug testing and policy have described what they believe to be the requisite elements of an effective anti-doping policy. For example, speaking at a Senate committee hearing in 2004, the Chief Executive Officer of USADA said such a policy:

> ... begins with a sample collection plan that includes appropriately timed, yearround, no-advance-notice testing. The plan must provide for the collection of samples at the time that athletes most benefit from doping and must be flexible and responsive to evolving doping techniques.

> ... must be built around a comprehensive list of categories of prohibited substances and methods .... programs must incorporate sufficient flexibility to deal with the creation and use of 'designer drugs' .... Therefore, the continued dedication of resources to the testing laboratories that are charged with developing and validating testing methods for this wide array of substances is an important aspect of deterrence.
>
> ... also combines defined sanctions of sufficient magnitude to deter drug use with a fair means of imposing such sanctions .... Significantly, while USADA believes the privacy rights of individuals accused of a doping violation must be respected, no individual's right should outweigh the rights of all athletes to compete in clean sport and to be assured that those who break the rules are appropriately sanctioned. ...
>
> [provides for] the education of athletes as to why healthy competition is important and why taking the uninformed health risks associated with prohibited substances is a bad choice. The achievements in sports, like the achievements in life, should be the result of hard work, commitment, and dedication.
>
> ... must devote significant resources to research for the detection of new doping substances and techniques and the pursuit of scientific excellence in doping control.[21]

Similarly, General Barry R. McCaffrey, U.S. Army (ret.), then-Director, Office of National Drug Control Policy, appeared at a Senate hearing in 1999 and stated that, with regard to international competition, the agency was focused on achieving these principles:

- A truly independent and accountable international anti-doping agency;
- Testing on a 365-day-a-year, no notice basis;
- No statute of limitations — whenever evidence becomes available that an athlete cheated by doping, the athlete will be stripped of his or her honors;
- Deterrence through the preservation of samples for at least 10 years — while a dishonest athlete may be able to defeat today's drug test, he or she has no way to know what will be detectable through tomorrow's scientific advances; and,
- Advanced research to end the present cat-and-mouse game of doping by closing the loopholes created by gaps in science.[22]

Conclusion

Combining elements of Madden's and McCaffrey's plans, such as a wellthought- out sample collection plan and a comprehensive list of prohibited substances, could result in an anti-doping program that would increase the probability of catching athletes who use prohibited substances, which, in turn, might also increase athletes' perceived risk of being caught. For example, requiring that samples be preserved for at least 10 years could aid in identifying athletes who have used performanceenhancing substances that were undetectable previously. As the investigation of the Bay Area Laboratory Co-Operative (BALCO) has shown, it is possible for individuals to develop what are known as designer steroids — substances that are advertised as providing effects similar to steroids, but are not identifiable by conventional laboratory tests.[23] A 10-year (or longer) retention period could help in closing this gap, particularly if it is accompanied by an aggressive research program aimed at detecting, and developing tests for, previously unknown substances. Also, imposing sanctions of sufficient magnitude and providing an education program on health risks could help to counterbalance incentives that might prompt athletes to use prohibited substances. Finally, establishment of an independent agency to manage testing, education, and research appears to be vital to a successful anti-doping program. It would seem desirable to place these functions in an organization independent from the organization that is responsible for supporting or employing athletes and that benefits directly, or even indirectly, from their performances.

While the anti-doping initiative of the Olympic movement includes many of these elements, it is uncertain whether major professional sports leagues in the United States, such as Major League Baseball and the NBA and NFL, are in a position to take similar steps. Public pressure and congressional interest may have played a role in prompting Major League Baseball and the players association to reopen their collective bargaining agreement in 2005 and modify the league's antidoping policy. One notable outcome was a change in the sanctions imposed on players caught using steroids.

Appendix

Table 2. Comparison of Selected Features of Major League Baseball's 2003-2004 Policy and 2005 Policy

	Major League Baseball MB) 2003-2004 Policy	Major League Baseball (MB) 2005 Policy (draft)a
— What organization or individual is responsible for administering the antidoping policy? — Is the organization or individual independent from the sponsoring organization(s)?	— Health Policy Advisory Committee (HPAC). — No. Major League Baseball and the Major League Baseball Players Association each select two members of the HPAC.	— HPAC. — No.
	Major League Baseball MB) 2003-2004 Policy	Major League Baseball (MB) 2005 Policy (draft)a
Are athletes tested for all prohibited substances?	No.[f]	No.[f]

Table 2. (Continued)

	Major League Baseball MB) 2003-2004 Policy	Major League Baseball (MB) 2005 Policy (draft)a
Does the anti-doping policy prohibit:		
— Steroidse	— Yes.	— Yes.
— Hormones and related substances	— Unclear.[l]	— Yes.[f]
— Beta-2 agonists	— Unclear.[l]	— Unclear.[l]
— Agents with antiestrogenic activity	— Unclear[l]	— Unclear.[l]
— Diuretics and other masking agents	— Yes.[i]	— Yes.[i]
— Enhancement of oxygen transfer	— No.	— No.
— Chemical and physical manipulation	— Yes.[i]	— Yes.[i]
— Gene doping	— No.	— No.
— Stimulants	— Unclear.[k]	— Unclear, except for ephedra, which is prohibited but not tested.[n,l]
— Glucocorticosteroids	— Unclear.[m]	— Unclear.[m]
Is a player responsible for what is in his body?	Unclear.[l]	No.
What laboratory tests the samples?	Subject is not addressed in the policy.	Subject is not addressed in the policy, but MB has indicated that testing is conducted at a WADAaccredited laboratory in Montreal.[q]
Are sanctions applicable to all prohibited substances?	No.[f]	No.[f]
What are the sanctions for testing positive for steroids?		
— First violation	— Played placed on clinical track (treatment program).	— 10-day suspension without pay.[q]
— Second violation	— 15-day suspension without pay or a maximum fine of $10,000.	— 30-day suspension without pay.
— Third violation	— 25-day suspension without pay or a maximum fine of $25,000.	— 60-day suspension without pay.
— Fourth violation	— 50-day suspension without pay or a maximum fine of $50,000.	— One-year suspension without pay.
— Fifth violation	— One-year suspension without pay or a maximum fine of $100,000.	— MB Commissioner imposes further discipline.
Is testing conducted during the off-season?	No.	Yes
What types of specimens are collected and tested?	Urine.	Urine.

Sources: Major League Baseball, *Major League Baseball's Joint Drug Prevention and Treatment Program*, n.d., p. 6, available at [http://reform. house.gov/Uploaded Files/031705%20MLB %20Policy. pdf]; Major League Baseball and Major League Baseball Players Association, *2003-2006 Basic Agreement*, n.d., available at [http://us.i1.yimg.com/ us.yimg.com/i/spo /mlbpa/mlbpa_cba.pdf].

Notes:

[a] The policy negotiated by Major League Baseball and the players association that takes effect during the 2005 season has not yet been ratified by the players, but apparently it is in effect. An article issued by *MLB.com* stated that an outfielder for the Tampa Bay Devil Rays tested positive for steroid use and, as a result, was suspended for the10 days. (Barry M. Bloom, "Rays' Sanchez Suspended for 10 Days," *MLB.com*, Apr. 3, 2005, available at [http://mlb.mlb.com/NASApp/ mlb/mlb/news/mlb_ search_archive.jsp].

[b] The federal government has established five schedules of controlled substances. The following three criteria are used to determine on which schedule to place a substance or drug: its potential for abuse, whether the item has a currently accepted medical use in the United States, and the probability that abuse of the substance could lead to physical or psychological dependence. Schedule I includes substances and drugs that have a high potential for abuse, that currently have no accepted medical use in the United States, and that lack accepted safety for use under medical supervision. Substances and drugs listed on one of the remaining four schedules have currently accepted medical uses, and the potential for abuse and the probability that abuse could lead to physical or psychological dependence declines from Schedule II through Schedule IV. (21 U.S.C. § 812(a) and (b).) Major League Baseball's list of prohibited substances includes drugs of abuse (cocaine, LSD, marijuana, opiates, Ecstasy, GHB, PCP, all drugs or substances listed on Schedule II, and all Schedule I drugs listed on Addendum C of the league's anti-doping policy) and all anabolic androgenic steroids listed on Schedule III. Section 3.C. of this policy explicitly excludes drugs of abuse from the testing program: "Except as set forth in Section 3.D. [reasonable cause testing], Players shall not be subject to either Survey or Program Testing for the use of any Drug of Abuse." (Major League Baseball and Major League Baseball Players Association, *2003-2006 Basic Agreement*, n.d., pp. 159-160, 163, available online at [http://us.i1.yimg. com/us.yimg. com/i/spo /mlbpa/mlbpa_cba.pdf].)

[c] The federal government has established five schedules of controlled substances. The following three criteria are used to determine on which schedule to place a substance or drug: its potential for abuse, whether the item has a currently accepted medical use in the United States, and the probability that abuse of the substance could lead to physical or psychological dependence. Schedule I includes substances and drugs that have a high potential for abuse, that currently have no accepted medical use in the United States, and that lack accepted safety for use under medical supervision. Substances and drugs listed on one of the remaining four schedules have currently accepted medical uses, and the potential for abuse and the probability that abuse could lead to physical or psychological dependence declines from Schedule II through Schedule IV. (21 U.S.C. § 812(a) and (b).) Major League Baseball's list of prohibited substances includes drugs of abuse (cocaine, LSD, marijuana, opiates, Ecstasy, GHB, PCP, ephedra, all drugs or substances listed on Schedule II, and all Schedule I drugs listed on Addendum B of the league's anti-doping policy) and all anabolic androgenic steroids listed on Schedule III. Section 3.B. of this policy explicitly excludes drugs of abuse from the testing program: "Except as set forth in Section 3.C. [reasonable cause testing], Players shall not be subject to testing for the use of any Drug of Abuse." (Major League Baseball, *Major League Baseball's Joint Drug Prevention and Treatment Program*, n.d., pp. 3 and 6, available at [http://reform.house.gov/Uploaded Files/ 031705% 20MLB % 20 Policy.pdf].)

[d] The use of the term "steroids" in this context refers to anabolic or anabolic androgenic steroids, substances which may help an athlete increase his or her muscle size and strength and re cover more quickly from injury. The class of substances known as "steroids" includes other types of substances. See "anabolic androgenic steroids" and "steroids" in the glossary.

e. The list of prohibited substances includes all of Schedule II and an extensive list of substances from Schedule I. It is unclear whether any substances known as "hormones" are listed on either of these schedules. Efforts to obtain clarification on this matter from Major League Baseball or the players association are continuing.

f. Human growth hormone (hGH) is on the list of prohibited substances, under the heading "steroids," but MB does not test for it. In testimony offered during a House Committee on Government Reform hearing, Robert D. Manfred Jr., Executive Vice President, MB, and Elliot J. Pellman, M.D., Medical Advisor to the Commissioner of Baseball, indicated that Major League Baseball does not test for human growth hormone (hGH). The rationale they offered was that no valid urine-based test exists. Mr. Manfred added: "Contrary to published reports, there is not an available, verified test for HGH, even with a blood sample." (U.S. Congress, House Committee on Government Reform, statements of Robert D. Manfred Jr., Executive Vice President, Major League Baseball, and Elliot J. Pellman, M.D., Medical Advisor to the Commissioner of Baseball, unpublished hearing, 109th Cong., 1st sess., Mar. 17, 2005, available online at [http://mlb.mlb.com |/NASApp /mlb/news/press_releases /intro.jsp] and [http://reform.house.gov/ Uploaded Files/ Pellman%20Testimony.pdf].) It should be noted that the World Anti-Doping Agency tested athletes for hGH at the 2004 Athens Olympics, using a blood test that had been developed and validated in partnership with the IOC and USADA. (World Anti Doping Agency, "Minutes of the WADA Executive Committee Meeting," Nov. 20, 2004, p. 20, at [http://www.wada-ama.org/en/ dynamic.ch2?pageCategory_id=44].)

g. The list of prohibited substances includes all of Schedule II and an extensive list of substances from Schedule I. It is unclear whether any substances known as "beta-2 agonists" are listed on either of these schedules. Efforts to obtain clarification on this matter from Major League Baseball or the players association are continuing.

h. The list of prohibited substances includes all of Schedule II and an extensive list of substances from Schedule I. It is unclear whether any substances known as "agents with anti-estrogenic activity" are listed on either of these schedules. Efforts to obtain clarification on this matter from Major League Baseball or the players association are continuing.

i. Masking substances (and methods) are not identified on the list of prohibited substances, but the policy states that any test will be considered "positive" if a player "attempts to substitute, dilute, mask, or adulterate a specimen sample or in any other manner alter a test." (Major League Baseball, *2003-2006 Basic Agreement*, p. 164.)

j. Masking substances (and methods) are not identified on the list of prohibited substances, but the policy states: "Attempts to substitute, dilute, mask, or adulterate a specimen sample are considered a positive test result." (Major League Baseball, *Major League Baseball's Joint Drug Prevention and Treatment Program*, p. 6.)

k. The list of prohibited substances includes all of Schedule II and an extensive list of substances from Schedule I. It is unclear whether any substances known as "stimulants" are listed on either of these schedules. Efforts to obtain clarification on this matter from Major League Baseball or the players association are continuing.

l. Ephedra is a prohibited substance, but it is not included in regular testing of players. (Major League Baseball, *Major League Baseball's Joint Drug Prevention and Treatment Program*, p. 3.) See footnote c. above.

m. The list of prohibited substances includes all of Schedule II and an extensive list of substances from Schedule I. It is unclear whether any substances known as "glucocorticosteroids" are listed on either of these schedules. Efforts to obtain clarification on this matter from Major League Baseball or the players association are continuing.

n. Absent an explicit statement about a player's responsibility for what is in his body, the following excerpt suggests that, depending upon the circumstances, a player's claim that a positive test resulted from a contaminated over-the-counter supplement could have been valid : "If ... a Player tests positive in the initial test for a Steroid and such positive test cannot be a result of a Player taking an over-the-counter supplement, the initial test shall be considered a positive result regardless of the outcome of the follow-up test."(Major League Baseball and Major League Baseball Players Association, *2003-2006 Basic Agreement*, p. 162.)

o. Major League Baseball and the players association agreed, in spring 2004, to have all drug testing under the *MB Joint Drug Prevention and Testing Program* conducted by the Doping Control Laboratory at the INRS-Instituted Armand-Flapper Research Center in Montreal. This is a WADA-accredited laboratory. (Major League Baseball, "MB Drug-Testing Programs Move to Olympic-Certified Laboratories," May 11, 2004, available at [http://mlb.mlb.com/NASApp/mlb/content/printer_friendly/mlb/y2004/m05/d11/c740823.jsp].)

p. Apparently, sanctions apply only to positive tests for steroids. As noted above, testing for other substances and drugs prohibited by the league will not be done as part of its ongoing testing program. Though players may be tested for these other substances when reasonable cause exists for doing so, no sanctions are included for positive tests of other substances.

q. The 2005 draft of MLB's anti-doping policy states that, for first through fourth violations, a fine may be levied in lieu of imposing a suspension. (Major League Baseball, *Major League Baseball's Joint Drug Prevention and Treatment Program*, n.d., pp. 11-12.) However, as reported in the *Washington Post* on Mar. 21, 2005, both parties (MB and MLBPA) have agreed to eliminate fines, leaving suspensions as the only sanction. ("Agreement Reached to Drop Fines," *Washington Post*, Mar. 21, 2005, p. D5.)

Glossary

Agents with anti-estrogenic activity — An agent with anti-estrogenic activity blocks the conversion of testosterone to estrogens (female hormones), or prevents or minimizes the body's response to estrogens present in the body. A male athlete who uses steroids may ingest an agent with anti-estrogen activity to help mitigate against breast development resulting from steroid use.[24]

Anabolic androgenic steroids — "Anabolic-androgenic steroids [AAS] are synthetic derivatives of testosterone .... Testosterone itself is not effective when taken orally or by injection, because it is susceptible to relatively rapid breakdown by the liver. The chemical structure of testosterone has been modified by pharmaceutical companies and pharmacologists to surmount this problem."[25] "'Anabolic' refers to muscle-building, and 'androgenic' refers to increased masculine characteristics.[26] Using steroids may help an individual increase his or her muscle size and strength and recover more quickly from injury."[27] Also see "Steroids."

Analogues (analogs) — "[S]ubstances derived from the modification or alteration of the chemical structure of another substance while retaining a similar pharmacological effect."[28] For example, the chemical structure of a steroid analogue would differ from the structure of a steroid, but it would promote the development of muscle.

Beta-2 agonists — "Beta-agonists are bronchodilator medicines that open airways by relaxing the muscles around the airways that tighten during an asthma attack."[29] Some beta-2 agonists, when taken into the bloodstream, may help to increase "skeletal muscle mass and decrease body fat."[30]

Beta-blockers — "Beta-blockers are commonly used for heart disease to lower blood pressure and decrease the heart rate, and may be used to decrease fine motor tremor.[31] Athletes may use beta-blockers illegally to try to stop their hands and bodies from shaking while competing in precision sports that require accuracy, a calm state and/or a steady hand."[32]

Diuretics — "Diuretics remove the excess water from the body. They are used in sports where the athletes are categorized by their body weight....."[33] Sports that have weight classes include wrestling, boxing, judo, and weightlifting. Diuretics also aid in diluting an athlete's urine "so that the presence of performance-enhancing drugs, or their metabolic counterparts, cannot be detected."[34]

Doping control — "The process including test distribution planning, *Sample* collection and handling, laboratory analysis, results management, hearings and appeals."[35] ("Doping control" is a term specific to WADA and the international sports community to describe efforts to eliminate the use of prohibited performanceenhancing substances and methods from sport.)[36]

Enhancement of oxygen transfer — An athlete may increase his body's oxygen capacity either by "artificially enhancing the uptake, transport, or delivery of oxygen," such as through the ingestion of erythorpoietin (see below), or through blood doping.[37] Blood doping involves the administration of blood cells. "Two to four units (one unit corresponds to 450 ml [milliliters] of whole blood are collected from the individual ... [and then] three to five days before the competition [the blood is] infused [into the individual]."[38]

Ephedra — "Ephedra is a plant that contains the chemical ephedrine, a stimulant similar to amphetamines. Athletes may take an over-the-counter supplement containing ephedra to reduce physical fatigue, lose weight or improve mental alertness."[39]

Epitestosterone — Epitestosterone, which is a natural steroid, plays an important role in testing an individual for the presence of excess testosterone. The ratio of testosterone to epitestosterone (T/E) usually is 1:1. A ratio of 6:1 or higher generally is an indication of illegal supplementation of testosterone.[40] (However, the World Anti-Doping Agency lowered its T/E threshold to 4:1 in 2005.[41])

Erythropoietin (EPO) — EPO, which is an alternative to blood doping, stimulates red blood cell production. It increases an individual's aerobic power by increasing the number of his or her red blood cells to "unnatural levels."[42]

Gene doping — "The non-therapeutic use of genes, genetic elements or of the modulation of gene expression, having the capacity to enhance athletic performance ....[43] This includes attempts to modulate hormonal control of production of normal substances in the body, such as growth hormone or erythropoietin."[44]

Glucocorticosteroids — "Glucocorticosteroids are powerful anti-inflammatory agents, [45] [which] affect the metabolism, and athletes may use them to get more energy."[46] Glucocorticosteroids are also known as glucocorticoids.

Human chorionic gonadotropin (hCG) — In males, hCG helps to stimulate the production of male hormones such as testosterone.[47] Male athletes may take hCG "to increase the ability of their body to produce testosterone and to prevent atrophy of the testicles that results from taking large doses of anabolic steroids."[48]

Human growth hormone (hGH) — HGH is "the hormone ... responsible for growth and when administered to an adult whose growth has stopped increases protein synthesis."[49] Athletes might use it to "induce anabolic effects, reduce muscle cell breakdown and reduce body fat."[50]

Insulin — Insulin is used by individuals who have diabetes to manage their blood sugar levels. Some athletes may use insulin in an effort "to increase muscle growth and improve muscle definition."[51]

Masking agents — "Substances that are used to prevent the detection of other substances or methods used by an athlete in doping. An example would be the attempt to change the pH of the urine to enhance excretion of a doping substance."[52]

Mimetics — Synthetic compounds "that produce the same (or a very similar effect) as another (especially a naturally occurring) compound."[53]

Pharmacological, chemical, and physical manipulation — "Pharmacological, chemical and physical manipulation is the *Use* of substances and methods, including masking agents, which alter, attempt to alter or may reasonably be expected to alter the integrity and validity of specimens collected in doping controls. These include but are not limited to catheterization, urine substitution and/or tampering, inhibition of renal excretion and alterations of testosterone and epitestosterone concentrations."[54] Manipulation may include "the addition of chemicals or other contaminants to the actual specimen following collection, with the intent of preventing the detection of a doping substance ...."[55] (This is an illustrative description. The actual substances and methods considered to constitute manipulation may vary from organization (or professional sports league) to organization.)

Precursor — "Steroid precursors are substances that are converted in the body into steroids ...."[56]

Prohormone — "A natural precursor of a hormone;[57] any substance that can be converted into a hormone."[58]

Steroids — "A class of compounds with common elements of their chemical structures, but wide ranging effects. *Androgenic-anabolic steroids* are the hormones responsible for secondary male sex characteristics; *estrogens* are the hormones responsible for development and maintenance of female secondary sex characteristics; *glucocorticosteroids* regulate carbohydrate, fat and protein metabolism; *mineralocorticoids* regulate the balance of water and electrolytes. In addition, steroids have been used for a variety of medical purposes, including reducing inflammation."[59] Also see "anabolic androgenic steroids."

Stimulants — "Stimulants are substances that act directly on the central nervous system to speed up parts of the brain and body."[60] Stimulants "can reduce fatigue, suppress appetite, and increase alertness and aggressiveness."[61]

Testosterone — "Testosterone is the main male hormone that maintains muscle mass and strength ...."[62]

References

[1] Charles E. Yesalis, William A. Anderson, William E. Buckley, and James E. Wright, *Incidence of the Nonmedical Use of Anabolic-Androgenic Steroids*, research monograph 102, U.S. Dept. of Health and Human Services, National Institute on Drug Abuse (Washington: GPO, 1990), pp. 97-98; Charles E. Yesalis and Michael S. Bahrke, "History of Doping in Sport," in *Performance-Enhancing Substances in Sport and Exercise*, Michael S. Bahrke and Charles E. Yesalis, eds. (Champaign, IL: Human Kinetics, 2002), pp. 1-2.

[2] Yesalis and Bahrke, "History of Doping in Sport," p. 1. (Italics in original.)

[3] World Anti-Doping Agency, "A Brief History of Anti-Doping," n.d., available online at [http://www.wada-ama.org/en/dynamic.ch2?page Category_id=20].

[4] Ibid., p. 2.

[5] U.S. Congress, House Committee on Government Reform, statement of Paul Tagliabue, Commissioner, National Football League, and Harold Henderson, Executive Vice President — Labor Relations, National Football League, unpublished hearing, 109th Cong., 1st. sess., Apr. 28, 2005, p. 5.

[6] Information provided by the NBA's Basketball Communications Office to the author on May 19, 2004.

[7] Efforts to obtain a copy of the National Hockey League's program, *NHL/NHLPA* [National Hockey League Players Association] *Substance Abuse and Behavioral Health Program* (SABHP) were unsuccessful. It is unclear whether this program includes performanceenhancing substances. This program took effect in September 1996 and apparently expired on September 15, 2004, when the collective bargaining agreement negotiated by the NHL and the players association expired.

[8] In 1999, the International Olympic Committee (IOC) convened a World Conference on Doping in Sport, which produced the Lausanne Declaration on Doping in Sport. The World Anti-Doping Agency (WADA) was established, pursuant to the Lausanne Declaration, on Nov. 10, 1999. (World Anti-Doping Agency, "WADA History," n.d., available at [http://www.wada-ama.org/en/dynamic.ch2?pageCategory_id=12].) The U.S. Anti-Doping Agency (USADA), which began operations Oct. 1, 2000, was created as a result of recommendations made by the U.S. Olympic Committee's Select Task Force on Externalization. It is responsible for anti-doping efforts within the U.S. Olympic movement. Specifically, USADA has the authority to test and educate U.S. Olympic, Paralympic, and Pan American athletes, adjudicate appeals, and conduct research in support of its antidoping efforts. (U.S. Anti-Doping Agency, "USADA History," n.d., available at [http://www.usantidoping.org/who/history.html]; U.S. Anti-Doping Agency, "USADA Mission," available at [http://www usantidoping. org/who/mission.html].) The Paralympics "are a multi-sport, multi-disability competition of elite, world-class, disabled athletes. Although similar in scope to the Olympic Games, the Paralympic Games provide an elite competition opportunity to athletes with a functional disability, which precludes their involvement in open competition of the Olympic Games." (U.S. Olympic Committee, "Paralympic Overview," n.d., available at [http://www.usoc.org/ education/paralympic_overview/paralympicindex.htm].) The Pan American Sports Organization (PAS) consists of 42 nations of Central, North, and South America, and the Caribbean. "The Pan American Games are held every four years just like the Olympic Games and precede the Games by a year. The Pan American Games consist of all summer Olympic sports, plus some non-Olympic sports, and serve as an Olympic-qualifying event for many of the participating sports." (U.S. Olympic Committee, "Pan American Games Overview," n.d., available at [http://www.olympic-usa.org/education/ panamoverview/ panindex.htm].)

[9] For example, the Olympic prohibition against beta-blockers applies to 18 sports (and only during competitions) including archery, curling, and gymnastics. (World Anti-Doping Agency, *The 2005 Prohibited List, International Standard*, n.d., available online at [http://www.wada-ama.org/rtecontent/document/list_book_2005_en.pdf], p. 18.)

[10] An athlete who has been banned under the WADA *Code* has been declared ineligible. An athlete's status during eligibility is as follows: "No Person who has been declared ineligible may, during the period of ineligibility, participate in any capacity in a Competition or activity (other than authorized anti-doping education or rehabilitation programs) authorized or organized by a Signatory or Signatory's member organization" (p. 35). Signatories are those organizations that have signed and agreed to comply with the WADA *Code* and include "the International Olympic Committee, International Federations, International Paralympic Committee, National Olympic Committees, National Paralympic Committees, Major Event Organizations, National Anti-Doping Organizations, and WADA." (World Anti-Doping Agency, *World Anti-Doping Code*, pp. 35, 75.) For example, the list of organizations that have accepted the WADA *Code* includes the International Fencing Federation, International Swimming Federation, International Tennis Federation, and the International Wrestling Federation. (World Anti-Doping Agency, "List of Sports Organizations Who Have Accepted the Code," n.d., available at [http://www.wadaama. org/en/print.asp?p=42255].)

[11] The federal government has established five schedules of controlled substances. The following three criteria are used to determine on which schedule to place a substance or drug: its potential for abuse, whether the item has a currently accepted medical use in the United States, and the probability that abuse of the substance could lead to physical or psychological dependence. Schedule I includes substances and drugs that have a high potential for abuse, that currently have no accepted medical use in the United States, and that lack accepted safety for use under medical supervision. Substances and drugs listed on one of the remaining four schedules have currently accepted medical uses, and the potential for abuse and the probability that abuse could lead to physical or psychological dependence declines from Schedule II through Schedule IV. (21 U.S.C. § 812(a) and (b).)

[12] R. Craig Kammerer, "Drug Testing in Sport and Exercise," in *Performance-Enhancing Substances in Sport and Exercise*, p. 330.

[13] In early summer 2003, USADA received a syringe from an individual who claimed to be a track and field coach. The then-anonymous coach also provided the names of American and international athletes that he alleged had used an undetectable steroid. USADA forwarded the contents of the syringe to the UCLA Olympic Analytic Laboratory, a WADAaccredited laboratory, for analysis. Dr. Don Catlin, head of the laboratory, determined that the substance was a designer steroid, meaning that it could not be detected by normal laboratory testing. The UCLA laboratory determined that the substance was tetrahydrogestrinone (THG) and developed a test for THG. (U.S. Anti-Doping Agency, "U.S. Anti-Doping Statement on Doping Case with Designer Steroids," press release, Oct. 16, 2003, available at [http://www. usantidoping. org/files/active/ resources/press_releases/ PressRelease_10_16_2003.pdf].) USADA

has alleged that the source of THG was the Area Laboratory Co-Operative (BALCO), which is located in Burlingame, CA. Internal Revenue Service agents raided BALCO in September 2003. (Mark Asher, "Bonds to Testify on Supplement Supplier," *Washington Post*, Oct. 22, 2003, p. D2.) As reported by the *Washington Post*, the Department of Justice initiated an investigation of BALCO in 2003, and the Senate Committee on Commerce requested and received information from the department's investigation. (Amy Shipley, "Olympic Officials to Request Federal Files," *Washington Post*, May 5, 2004, p. D9; Amy Shipley, "USADA Bans White for 2 Years," *Washington Post*, May 202, 2004, p. D5.)

[14] Maske and Shapiro, "NFL Strengthens Steroid Policy," p. D8.

[15] Major League Baseball, *Major League Baseball's Joint Drug Prevention and Treatment Program*, n.d., pp. 3 and 6, available at [http://reform. house.gov/ UploadedFiles/ 031705%20MLB%20Policy.pdf]. See *Table 1* for additional information. Major League Baseball's policy states: "In the event that any HPAC [Health Policy Advisory Committee] member has information that gives him/her reasonable cause to believe that a Player has, in the previous 12-month period, engaged in the use, possession, sale or distribution of a Prohibited Substance, such member shall immediately request a meeting (or conference call) to present such information to the other HPAC members. If HPAC agress bya majority vote that such reasonable cause exists, the Player will be subejct to immediate testing ...." (Major League Baseball, *Major League Baseball's Joint Drug Prevention and Treatment Program*, n.d., p. 6, available at [http://reform.house.gov/UploadedFiles/031705%20MLB%20Policy .pdf].)

[16] Major League Baseball, *Major League Baseball's Joint Drug Prevention and Treatment Program*, n.d., pp. 11-12.

[17] R. Craig Kammerer, "Drug Testing in Sport and Exercise," in *Performance-Enhancing Substances in Sport and Exercise*, pp. 330-331. As noted below (**Table 1**, footnote g.), a blood-based test for human growth hormone has been developed.

[18] World Anti-Doping Agency, *World Anti-Doping Code*, 2003, available online at [http://www.wada-ama. org/ rtecontent/document/code_v3.pdf], p. 1.

[19] Ibid., p. 3.

[20] National Football League, *National Football League Policy on Anabolic Steroids and Related Substances*, 2003 (as amended May 15, 2003), p. 1.

[21] U.S. Congress, Senate Committee on Commerce, Science and Transportation, *Steroid Use in Professional and Amateur Sports*, Mar. 10, 2004, 108th Cong., 2nd sess., statement of Terry Madden, Chief Executive Officer, United States Anti-Doping Agency, unpublished, available at [http://commerce.senate. gov/hearings/witnesslist. cfm?id= 1100].

[22] U.S. Congress, Senate Committee on Commerce, Science, and Transportation, *Effects of Performance Enhancing Drugs on the Health of Athletes and Athletic Competition*, 106th Cong., 1st sess., Oct. 20, 1999 (Washington: GPO, 2002), p. 21.

[23] Steve Fawner, "A Search for Truth in Substance," *Washington Post*, Dec. 4, 2003, pp. D1, D10.

[24] U.S. Anti-Doping Agency, *2005 Guide to Prohibited Substances and Prohibited Methods of Doping*, p. 25; William N. Taylor, *Anabolic Steroids and the Athlete*, 2nd ed. (Jefferson, NC: McFarland and Co., 2002), p. 35.
[25] Michael S. Bahrke and Charles E. Yesalis, "Anabolics," in *Performance-Enhancing Substances in Sport and Exercise*, p. 33.
[26] National Institutes of Health, National Institute on Drug Abuse, "NIDA InfoFacts: Steroids (Anabolic-Androgenic)," n.d., available at [http://www.nida.nih.gov/Infofax /steroids.html].
[27] U.S. Anti-Doping Agency, "Medical," n.d., available at [http://www.usantidoping.org/ resources/glossary/medical.aspx].
[28] Australian Sports Drug Agency, "Fact Sheet: Hormones and Related Substances," n.d., available at [http://www.asda.org.au/athletes/sub_fact_sheets/hormones.htm].
[29] U.S. Anti-Doping Agency, "Medical."
[30] Australian Sports Drug Agency, "Fact Sheet: Beta-2 Agonists," n.d., available at [http://www.asda.org.au/athletes/sub_fact_sheets/beta2.htm]; Gordon S. Lynch, "Beta-2 Agonists," in *Performance-Enhancing Substances in Sport and Exercise*, p. 47.
[31] U.S. Anti-Doping Agency, "Medical."
[32] Australian Sports Drug Agency, "Fact Sheet: Beta Blockers," n.d., available at [http://www.asda.org.au/athletes/sub_fact_sheets/beta.htm].
[33] U.S. Anti-Doping Agency, "Medical."
[34] Lawrence E. Armstrong, "Diuretics," in *Performance-Enhancing Substances in Sport and Exercise*, p. 111.
[35] World Anti-Doping Agency, *International Standard for Testing*, p. 8.
[36] Information provided electronically by the U.S. Anti-Doping Agency to the author on Apr. 8, 2005.
[37] U.S. Anti-Doping Agency, *2005 Guide to Prohibited Substances and Prohibited Methods of Doping*, 2004, p. 10, available at [http://www.usantidoping. org/athletes /downloads .aspx?cid=2].
[38] Björn T. Ekblom, "Blood Doping," in *Performance-Enhancing Substances in Sport and Exercise*, pp. 94-95; U.S. Anti-Doping Agency, "Medical."
[39] Mayo Clinic, "Teen Athletes and Performance-Enhancing Substances: What Parents Can Do," Dec. 22, 2004, available at [http://www.mayoclinic. com/involke.cfm?id= SM00045].
[40] R. Craig Kammerer, "Drug Testing in Sport and Exercise," in *Performance-Enhancing Substances in Sport and Exercise*, p. 328.
[41] World Anti-Doping Agency, *The 2005 Prohibited List International Standard*, n.d., p. 7, available at [http://www.wada-ama.org/en/dynamic.ch2?pageCategory_id=174].
[42] National Center on Addiction and Substance Abuse at Columbia University, *Winning at Any Cost: Doping in Olympic Sports*, Sept. 2000 (New York: Columbia University), pp. 24- 25; U.S. Anti-Doping Agency, *2005 Guide to Prohibited Substances and Prohibited Methods of Doping*, p. 49.
[43] U.S. Anti-Doping Agency, *2005 Guide to Prohibited Substances and Prohibited Methods of Doping*, p. 10.
[44] Ibid., p. 29.

[45] Australian Sports Drug Agency, "Fact Sheet: Glucocorticosteroids," n.d., avaialble at [http://www.asda.org.au/athletes/sub_fact_sheets/glucocorticosteroids.htm].
[46] Information provided electronically by the U.S. Anti-Doping Agency to the author on Apr. 1, 2005.
[47] U.S. National Library of Medicine and National Institutes of Health, Medline Plus, "Drug Information: Chorionic Gonadotropin (Systemic)," Jan. 21, 2004, available at [http://www.nlm.nih.gov/ medlineplus/druginfo/uspdi/202266.html].
[48] Cynthia Kuhn, Scott Swartzwelder, and Wilkie Wilson, *Pumped* (New York: W.W. Norton and Co., 2000), p. 83.
[49] U.S. Anti-Doping Agency, *2005 Guide to Prohibited Substances and Prohibited Methods of Doping*, p. 49.
[50] Australian Sports Drug Agency, "Fact Sheet: Human Growth Hormone (hGH)," n.d., available at [http://www.asda.org.au/athletes/sub_fact_sheets/human.htm].
[51] Australian Sports Drug Agency, "Fact Sheet: Insulin," available at [http://www.asda.org.au/athletes/sub_fact_sheets/insulin.htm].
[52] U.S. Anti-Doping Agency, *2005 Guide to Prohibited Substances and Prohibited Methods of Doping*, p. 26.
[53] *Oxford English Dictionary Online*, available at [http://dictionary.oed.com].
[54] U.S. Anti-Doping Agency, *2004 United States Anti-Doping Agency Guide to Prohibited Substances and Prohibited Methods of Doping*, 2003, p. 19. (Italics in original.)
[55] U.S. Anti-Doping Agency, *2005 Guide to Prohibited Substances and Prohibited Methods of Doping*, 2004, p. 26.
[56] U.S. Olympic Committee, "USA Luge Joins Coalition Formed to Support Dietary Supplement Regulation," press release, Apr. 24, 2003, available online at [http://www.usolympicteam.com/73_8410.htm].
[57] *Oxford English Dictionary Online*, available at [http://dictionary.oed.com].
[58] *Dorland's Illustrated Medical Dictionary.*
[59] Information provided electronically by the U.S. Anti-Doping Agency to the author on Apr. 8, 2005. (Italics in original.)
[60] Australian Sports Drug Agency, "Fact Sheet: Stimulants," n.d., available at [http://www.asda.org.au/athletes/sub_fact_sheets/stimulants.htm].
[61] Mayo Clinic, "Performance-Enhancing Drugs: Dangerous, Damaging and Potentially Deadly."
[62] Mayo Clinic, "Testosterone Therapy: The Answer for Aging Men?" Apr. 13, 2004, available at [http://www.mayoclinic.com/invoke.cfm?id=MC00030].

In: Hot Topics in Sports and Athletics
Editor: Samuel R. Bakere, pp. 115-127

ISBN 978-1-60456-077-0

Chapter 7

Validity of the Brunel Mood Scale for Use with UK, Italian and Hungarian Athletes

Andrew M. Lane[1*], Istvan Soos[2], Eva Leibinger[3], Istvan Karsai[4] and Pal Hamar[3]
[1]University of Wolverhampton, UK
[2]University of Sunderland, UK
[3]Semmeilweis University, Budapest
[4]University of Pecs, Hungary

Abstract

The present study investigated the factorial validity of the Brunel Mood Scale for use with UK, Italian and Hungarian athletes. One thousand five hundred and eleven mood responses from athletes were analysed using Confirmatory Factor Analysis (CFA). CFA on the Italian, Hungarian and UK athletes were close to the .90 criterion for acceptable fit initially highlighted by Bentler (1990), but below the .95 fit index suggested by Hu and Bentler (1995). It is argued that CFA results lend some support for the proposed validity of an eight-factor and 32-item mood scale. However, as the fit index was marginal, further work was needed. Eight separate CFAs on each subscale indicated acceptable fit indices for each factor. As confusion is a cognitive rather than affective construct, we decided to remove confusion and re-analyse data on a 21-item and seven-factor scale. CFA results on the 21-item and seven-factor scale indicated fit indices over .90, hence an improvement over the 32-item version. In conclusion, the 21-item and 32-item BRUMS represent a theoretically and empirically supported approach to investigating mood for use in UK, Hungarian and Italian athletes.

* A.M.Lane2@wlv.ac.uk.

Introduction

Demonstrating validity is fundamental to theory testing. Valid and reliable measures provide the backbone for assessing constructs whether it is for research or practice. Schutz (1994) emphasized the importance of extending validity to a different population. The inextricable link between theory testing and construct measurement suggests that thorough investigation of the validity of measures should be the first stages in the research process.

In a review of mood measures, Lane (2004) argued that one of the most prominent tools used to assess emotion and mood in sport psychology has been the Profile of Mood States (POMS: McNair, Lorr, and Droppleman, 1971, 1992). He acknowledged that the POMS has numerous limitations, one being that it was developed and validated for use in a clinical population and that it has a markedly unpleasant orientation. This said, the POMS is still a commonly used scale in research and practice alike. The POMS is proposed to assess six mood states: anger, confusion, depression, fatigue, tension, and vigour. A rigorous validation program of the 24-item Brunel Mood Scale for use with athletes has been conducted (Terry, Lane, Lane, and Keohane, 1999; Terry, Lane, and Fogarty, 2003). Face validity was developed over two stages involving samples of adolescents who rated the comprehensibility of items. Participants rated the extent to which items in the pool assessed the six mood states assessed in the POMS. They also assessed the relative ease in which participants could understand the meaning of the items. In 1999, Terry and colleagues argued that this work was fundamental to the validation program as a limitation of the POMS is that participants do not readily understand many items. Examples to illustrate this point include items such as 'Blue' and 'Grovely'. By starting the validation procedure with adolescents, this ensured that the level of education of participants would not restrict the generalizability of the measure. In addition, by starting with adolescents, this increases the likelihood that most participants would find items easy to understand, and therefore, reduce completion time. Completion time is a important concern for researchers interested in assessing mood states before competition, or any other achievement related context such as before an examination or before a job interview.

Given the proposal that validity is fundamental to theory testing it is important to describe the procedure used by Terry and colleagues in the development and validation of their scale. Terry et al. (1999, 2003) used confirmatory factor analysis to produce a 24-item 6-factor measure. The study conducted in 2003 confirmed factorial validity across different sample by using multisample confirmatory factor analysis. Results showed factorial invariance between items and factors and between factors across different four disparate samples. It is important to recognise the contribution of these studies to the literature as few questionnaires have been subjected to such rigorous tests. Terry et al. demonstrated that the relationship between the item and factor is consistent between different samples. Previous research has conducted confirmatory factor analyses on different samples and suggested that acceptable fit indices show factorial invariance. This is not necessarily the case as there can be subtle differences between samples that are not noticed simply because the researcher has not tested to find these differences. For example, an item might show a strong relationship with a factor in one study but a weak relationship in another study. If, for example, we find support for the integrity of the depression scale among athletes and students in two separate confirmatory factor analyses, we could tentatively assume support for the integrity of the scale between samples. However, we should test the extent to which items and factors are invariant before such a claim can be verified. It could be that there is a difference in the size of relationships between some items. For example, if the item 'downhearted' has a strong relationship (r = .80 for instance) with depressed mood among athletes but a weaker relationship among students (r = .5 for instance), this suggests that downhearted has a more prominent influence in the construct among athletes. Arguably, such a finding shows that there subtle differences between nature of the factor between different samples. The results of Terry et al that demonstrate factorial invariance represent an important step forward with regards to confirming the validity of the BRUMS.

Criterion validity is a second aspect of validity and tested by examining correlations between the target construct measured on one scale with the same target construct measured on a separate scale. Terry et al. (1999, 2003) tested the criterion validity of scales on the BRUMS through relationships with the PANAS (Watson, Clark, and Tellegen, 1988) and the State Anger-Expression Inventory (STAXI; Spielberger, 1991). Relationships were consistent with theoretical predictions, thereby providing evidence of criterion validity. Whilst this evidence provides support for the supposed validity of the BRUMS, it should be noted that there are several similarities between the scales. For example, there are shared items in the BRUMS and the PANAS. Participants reporting 'nervous' on one questionnaire should logically provide the same score on the second scale when the two scales are administered simultaneously. This is particularly pertinent for the BRUMS and PANAS as both are single adjective checklists. The STAXI differs and BRUMS should correlate as both are configured to a certain extent around the term 'angry'.

A limitation of the BRUMS that Lane (2004) recognised is that vigour is only positive mood construct assesses. Recent research has extended validation of the scale to include a calmness factor and a happiness factor (Lane and Jarrett, 2005) to produce a 32-item and eight-factor scale. The subscales of happiness and calmness were taken from the UWIST (Matthews, Jones, and Chamberlain, 1990). Eight mood dimensions are proposed to provide a more balanced assessment of positive mood and negative mood.

The purpose of the present study was to investigate the factorial validity of the 32-items BRUMS for use with UK, Hungarian and Italian students. As applied work tends to require participants to complete measures in conditions where brevity is paramount, a second purpose was to develop psychometrically measure with 3-items per factor. When considering developing external validity, Lane, Lane, and Matheson (2004) proposed that a researcher should select one of three options available. One option is to use a previously validated inventory on the new population and assume validity, and therefore conduct only a few validation checks. A second option is to cross-validate the measure. A third option is to develop a new measure from principles. Previous research has tended to use the first option (Schutz, 1994). If researchers are to use self-report measures to test theoretical links, the first step in this process should be to demonstrate the validity of measures used. We suggest that the second option should be conducted as a minimum requirement, and it is with this thought in mind that drives the present study.

Method

Translation from English to Italian and Hungarian

The second author translated the 32-item measure from English into Hungarian. Two experts at the Physical Education and Sports Science Faculty, Semmeilweis University, Budapest, Hungary checked for accuracy and comprehensibility. It was further checked by an expert at the Institute of Physical Education and Sport Sciences, University of Pecs, Hungary. The questionnaire was translated into Italian using a similar procedure.

Participants

UK athletes were 664 (Male, N = 416; Female, N = 248: Age: M = 21.11, SD = 3.44). There were 540 responses from Italian athletes (Age: M = 20.01, SD = 3.01) and 307 responses from Hungarian athletes (Age: M = 20.09, SD = 2.98). Participants completed mood measures retrospectively before performance perceived as successful and a performance perceived unsuccessful.

Data Analysis

Following the recommendations of Byrne (2000), the hypothesized 32-item, eight-factor model of mood was first tested on each sample. Confirmatory factor analysis (CFA) using EQS V7 (Bentler and Wu, 1995) was used to test the model, which specified that items were related to their hypothesised factor with the variance of the factor fixed at 1. Consistent with theoretical predictions and previous empirical support, the latent factors anger, calmness, confusion, depression, fatigue, happiness, tension and vigour were allowed to correlate.

The choice of cut-off criteria used to evaluate model adequacy is a contentious issue. Some researchers favour a two-index strategy, with the indices selected on the basis of sample size, model complexity, and the distributional properties of the data (Hu and Bentler, 1999). We followed the approach of Byrne (1998, 2000) and Hoyle and Panter (1995).

Two incremental fit indices were used; the Comparative Fit Index (CFI: Bentler, 1990) and the non-normed fit index or Tucker-Lewis index (TLI: Tucker and Lewis, 1973). Incremental fit indices are based on comparisons between the hypothesised model and a null model (in which there are no relationships among the observed variables) and are not influenced by sample size. Kline (1998) proposed that values for the CFI and TLI of less than .90 indicate that the hypothesized model could be substantially improved, whereas Hu and Bentler (1999) suggested that, in most circumstances, values should approach .95. The fourth index used was the Root Mean Square Error of Approximation (RMSEA: Steiger, 1990), which indicates the mean discrepancy between the observed covariances and those implied by the model per degree of freedom, and therefore has the advantage of being sensitive to model complexity. A value of .05 or lower indicates a good fit and values up to .08 indicate an acceptable fit (Browne and Cudeck, 1993). Byrne (1998) described the RMSEA as "one of the most informative criteria in structural equation modelling" (p. 112).

Results

Multivariate kurtosis indicated that assumptions of normal distributed were violated among Hungarian students (Mardia's coefficient = 197.39; Normalized Estimate = 37.07), Italian (Mardia's Coefficient = 241.40; Normalized Estimate = 60.13). Data were estimated using the ROBUST with the maximum likelihood estimation method.

CFA on the Italian, Hungarian and UK athletes are contained in Table 1. As Table 1 indicates, fit indices were close to the .90 criterion for acceptable fit initially highlighted by Bentler (1990), but below the .95 fit suggested by Hu and Bentler (1995). The RMSEA for all models was below .10 and therefore indicative of acceptable model fit. Factor loadings for the measure for each nationality are contained in Table 2. As Table 2 indicates, factor loadings were generally consistent across nationalities. There were inconsistent factor loadings for the items anxious, calm, composed, confused, exhausted, mixed-up, nervous, sleepy, and tired.

Relationships between mood states in each Nationality are contained in Table 3. Relationships between all pleasant mood states were all significant and positive. Vigour was more strongly related to happiness than to calmness in each nationality with especially large relationships among Italian athletes. Relationships between unpleasant mood states were all significant among Italian and Hungarian athletes. The general trend of significant relationships among unpleasant mood states was supported for UK athletes other than weak relationships between anger and fatigue, anger and tension, and tension and fatigue.

Table 1. CFA results for the 8-factor 32-item model of mood among Hungarian, Italian and UK Students

	Hungary	Italy	Mood All
Bentler-Bonett Normed Fit Index	.89	.89	.90
Bentler-Bonett Non-Normed Fit Index	.89	.86	.90
Robust Comparative Fit Index (RCFI)	.90	.90	.92
Root Mean-Square Error of Approximation (RMSEA)	.07	.07	.06
90% Confidence Interval of RMSEA	.06-.07	.07-.07	.06-.07

Table 2. Standardised factor loadings for the 32-item scale among Hungarian, Italian and UK athletes

Items	Factor loading	R^2	Factor loading	R^2	Factor loading	R^2
	Hungarian		Italian		UK	
Active	.89	.79	.79	63	.82	.68
Alert	.89	.80	.78	61	.79	.63
Angry	.76	.58	.69	49	.88	.78
Annoyed	.77	.59	.80	64	.88	.77
Anxious	.67	.45	.54	30	.86	.74
Bad tempered	.87	.76	.84	71	.87	.76
Bitter	.82	.67	.87	.75	.80	.65
Calm	.68	.47	.67	.45	.74	.55
Cheerful	.87	.76	.80	.64	.81	.66
Composed	.81	.65	.42	.18	.65	.43
Confused	.53	.28	.69	.48	.71	.50
Contented	.77	.59	.81	.66	.62	.39
Depressed	.81	.66	.75	.56	.84	.70
Downhearted	.71	.51	.77	.60	.83	.69
Energetic	.82	.68	.87	.75	.85	.73
Exhausted	.78	.61	.55	.30	.75	.56
Happy	.78	.61	.82	.67	.84	.70
Lively	.77	.59	.80	.64	.79	.63
Miserable	.72	.51	.83	.70	.79	.63
Nervous	.74	.55	.55	.31	.90	.81
Panicky	.72	.53	.70	.49	.81	.65
Relaxed	.70	.49	.76	.57	.83	.69
Restful	.62	.39	.72	.52	.62	.38
Satisfied	.69	.48	.79	.62	.71	.50
Sleepy	.69	.48	.59	.35	.81	.67
Tired	.84	.71	.60	.36	.92	.85
Uncertain	.75	.56	.76	.58	.70	.49
Unhappy	.73	.54	.84	.71	.84	.71
Worn-out	.85	.72	.74	.55	.82	.68
Worried	.78	.61	.74	.55	.79	.62
Mixed-up	.50	.25	.79	.63	.89	.80
Muddled	.79	.63	.71	.51	.92	.84

Table 3. Factor correlations among mood states among Hungarian athletes (all correlations are significant at p < .05)

	Vigour	Calmness	Happiness	Anger	Depression	Tension	Fatigue
Hungarian							
Calmness	.51						
Italian	.67						
UK	.43						
Happiness							
Calmness	.79	.75					
Italian	.94	.77					
UK	.67	.81					
Anger							
Calmness	-.62	-.44	-.64				
Italian	-.54	-.39	-.58				
UK	-.13	-.22	-.37				
Depression							
Calmness	-.60	-.35	-.62	.93			
Italian	-.65	-.48	-.65	.89			
UK	-.37	-.37	-.57	.75			
Tension							
Calmness	-.35	-.64	-.55	.64	.68		
Italian	-.44	-.71	-.45	.52	.61		
UK	.05	-.41	-.38	.33	.43		
Fatigue							
Calmness	-.46	-.37	-.48	.58	.71	.68	
Italian	-.55	-.50	-.47	.78	.88	.87	
UK	-.55	-.18	-.28	.27	.37	-.07	
Confusion							
Calmness	-.47	-.51	-.60	.69	.80	.99	.76
Italian	-.63	-.66	-.64	.63	.75	.94	.90
UK	-.27	-.38	-.46	.53	.74	.69	.25

Conclusion

CFA findings lend some support for the proposed validity of an eight-factor and 32-item mood scale. However, marginal fit indices, inconsistent factor loadings and relationships between mood states suggest further that work is needed. Therefore, the decision was to analyse each factor independently. This type of analysis provides some insight into the integrity of each mood state scale.

Confirmatory Factor Analysis on Each Mood State When Analysed Separately

The results of eight separate CFAs are contained in Table 4. Results for calmness, confusion, and depression showed acceptable fit indices. It should be noted that the RMSEA, which takes into account model complexity, tends to penalise simple models. With only 4-items in each mood state being analysed the models tested where simple. Therefore, it should not be too surprising that happiness, fatigue, tension and vigour showed acceptable fit indices for the NFI and CFI but poor indices for the RMSEA. The strategy was to use factor loadings to modify the questionnaire to produce a shortened scale.

Table 4. Confirmatory factor analysis for all mood states when analysed independently

	Anger	Calmness	Confusion	Depression	Fatigue	Happiness	Tension	Vigour
NFI	.94	.99	.99	.99	.97	.97	.99	.97
NNFI	.83	.97	.96	.97	.90	.92	.96	.90
CFI	.94	.99	.99	.99	.97	.98	.99	.97
RMSEA	.16	.07	.06	.06	.17	.13	.11	.19
90% Confidence intervals for RMSEA	.13-.18	.03-11	.03-.09	.03-.09	.14-.20	.10-.16	.09-.14	.16-.22

Factor loadings for each mood states are contained in Table 5. It should be stressed that these are the results of eight independent analyses. Anger demonstrated four items with moderate factor loadings, a result that somewhat contradicts summary fit indices which suggested a marginal fit. Factor loadings for other subscales indicated moderate to high factor loadings with all items showing acceptable values, findings that would be expected given the relatively high overall fit indices reported. The decision was made to remove the weakest loading item from each subscale and re-analyse data. A further decision was to remove confusion as a mood state.

It is highly questionable whether confusion is a mood state. The items 'confused, mixed-up, muddled and uncertain' are flavoured with cognitive rather than affective expression. Recent research removed confusion from a mood-regulation measure (Hewston, Lane, Karageorghis, and Nevill, 2005) for similar reasons. Beedie (2005) argued that confusion was not a mood state but a symptom of mood disorder. Beedie also raised an important question. He asked 'what mood states are relevant to sport? – confusion is not likely to be one of these subscales. Confusion items rarely appear in the items generated in Hanin's (2000) research. Recent research that developed an emotion scale for use in sport (Jones, Lane, Bray, Uphill, and Catlin, 2005) only included anger, anxiety, dejection, happiness and excitement, hence they also are likely to argue that confusion is a consequence of anxiety. Given the above arguments and research evidence, we decided to remove confusion and re-analyse data on a 21-item and seven-factor scale.

Table 5. Factor loadings for each mood subscale

	Factor loading	Error variance	R^2
Anger			
Angry	.90	.43	.81
Annoyed	.88	.45	.79
Bad tempered	.86	.49	.75
Bitter	.80	.60	.64
Calmness			
Calm	.72	.68	.52
Composed	.61	.79	.37
Relaxed	.85	.52	.73
Restful	.63	.76	.40
Confusion			
Confused	.69	.71	.48
Uncertain	.66	.74	.44
Mixed-up	.89	.43	.80
Muddled	.94	.33	.88
Depression			
Depressed	.86	.50	.74
Downhearted	.84	.53	.71
Miserable	.80	.60	.64
Unhappy	.80	.59	.64
Fatigue			
Exhausted	.72	.68	.52
Sleepy	.80	.58	.65
Tired	.94	.32	.89
Worn-out	.81	.57	.66
Happiness			
Cheerful	.80	.58	.65
Contented	.60	.79	.36
Happy	.86	.51	.74
Satisfied	.69	.72	.47
Tension			
Anxious	.87	.49	.75
Nervous	.92	.38	.85
Panicky	.78	.61	.62
Worried	.75	.65	.57
Vigour			
Active	.86	.51	.73
Alert	.82	.57	.67
Energetic	.82	.56	.68
Lively	.75	.66	.56

The 21-Item Seven Factor Mood Scale

CFA results on the 21-item and seven-factor scale are contained in Table 6. Results show fit indices have a marginal improvement in comparison to the 32-item questionnaire. With reference to acceptable fit indices argued as needed for acceptable fit by Hu and Bentler (1995), all CFA and RMSEA results are acceptable. For the UK sample, NFI and NNFI results are on the .95 limit, however, Hungarian and Italian results are marginally below the threshold. Factor loadings for the 21-item questionnaire are contained in Table 7.

Table 6. Confirmatory factor analysis for the 21-item and seven-factor scale

	Hungary	Italy	UK
Bentler-Bonett Normed Fit Index	.92	.92	.95
Bentler-Bonett Non-Normed Fit Index	.92	.93	.95
Comparative Fit Index (CFI)	.95	.95	.95
Root Mean-Square Error of Approximation (RMSEA)	.08	.08	.06
90% Confidence Interval of RMSEA	069-086	.071-.082	.060-.066

Table 7. Factor loadings for each mood subscale for the 21-item seven-factor scale among Hungarian, Italian and UK athletes

	Hungarian athletes		Italian athletes		UK athletes	
Item	Factor loading	R^2	Factor loading	R^2	Factor loading	R^2
Active	.91	.84	.87	.75	.87	.76
Alert	.91	.83	.86	.74	.83	.70
Angry	.87	.75	.77	.59	.90	.82
Annoyed	.86	.75	.88	.77	.89	.80
Anxious	.76	.57	.68	.46	.87	.76
Bad-tempered	.79	.62	.79	.62	.84	.71
Calm	.69	.48	.69	.48	.75	.56
Cheerful	.90	.81	.80	.64	.83	.69
Composed	.80	.64	.41	.17	.67	.45
Depressed	.82	.68	.74	.54	.83	.69
Downhearted	.73	.54	.78	.62	.85	.72
Energetic	.78	.61	.82	.67	.80	.64
Happy	.80	.65	.79	.63	.85	.72
Nervous	.82	.68	.64	.41	.92	.85
Panicky	.66	.44	.67	.44	.77	.60
Relaxed	.69	.48	.69	.48	.79	.63
Satisfied	.67	.44	.76	.59	.68	.46
Sleepy	.72	.51	.65	.42	.81	.66
Tired	.86	.75	.62	.39	.95	.91
Unhappy	.72	.53	.81	.66	.82	.67
Worn-out	.82	.68	.73	.54	.79	.63

General Discussion and Conclusions

The present study has addressed two issues. The first is the development of a seven-factor measure of mood, that although based on the POMS model, assesses a greater number of positive mood states. The second aim was to extend validity to non-English speaking participants. Recent research has demonstrated the use of mood state monitoring in the response to stressful situations (Soos, Leibinger, Karsai, and Hamar, in press), and as Soos, Leibinger et al. outlined that there is a need to identify the extent to which students experience unpleasant and dysfunctional mood states in sport students in countries across Europe. A validated scale for use with students who speak a different language to English would be suitable for such a purpose.

Findings from the present study lend support for both the 32-item and 21-item seven-factor models. This contrasts with recent research that has attempted to validated a mood measure among Hungarian student-athletes. Soos, Lane, Leibinger, Karsai, and Hamar (2005) reported poor factorial validity for the Profile of Mood States Short-Form (POMS-SF: Grove and Prapavessis, 1992) among Hungarian athletes. Soos, Lane et al. also proposed that the POMS offered a limited conceptualisation of positive mood and used the Grove and Prapavessis (1992) 40-item version of the POMS to assess the six original factors (anger, confusion, depression, fatigue, tension, and vigour) and an esteem-related aspect of mood. Although obtaining a large sample size ($N = 623$), results indicated poor factorial validity for the hypothesised seven-factor model. It is therefore suggested that both the 32-item and 21-item extended BRUMS provide a stronger measure than the POMS-SF for use with Hungarian students.

An issue labelled at mood research driven by the POMS is the extent to which mood states experienced by athletes are captured in the scale. Recent research has developed a measure of emotion grounded in the experience of athletes. Jones et al. (2005) followed equally rigorous procedures as Terry et al. (1999) in assessing the comprehensively and contextual relevance of items. In stage one, 264 athletes completed an open-ended questionnaire to identify emotions experienced in sport and in the second stage, 148 athletes verified the item pool. Jones et al. grouped this list of items under five constructs; anger, anxiety, dejection, excitement and happiness. Subsequent development of the Sport Emotion Questionnaire (SEQ) through confirmatory factor analysis found evidence in support for the scale. Concurrent validity of the SEQ was explored through investigating relationships with the 24-item BRUMS. It is the relationships between the BRUMS and SEQ provide the most intriguing findings. Results indicate high correlations between depression-dejection ($r = .87$), anxiety-tension ($r = .93$), and the two anger scales ($r = .94$). Moderate relationships were evidenced for excitement and vigour ($r = .85$) and happiness and vigour ($r = .69$). A weak significant relationship emerged for dejection and fatigue: $r = .24$. Therefore, although Jones et al. (2005) started from a qualitative base, the resultant measure converges with the BRUMS for anger, depression and tension, which arguably according to Lane and Terry (2000) represent the most powerful mood states.

Although there is evidence to support the validity of the POMS in sport, it will not be without its critics. It has a markedly unpleasant orientation even though the present study has sought to provide a more even balance of pleasant and unpleasant mood states. Beedie (2005) further criticised the POMS as confusion is a cognitive state, that is either a consequence or antecedent of a mood state; fatigue and vigour and physiological states rather than mood states. In conclusion, the 21-item and 32-item BRUMS represent a theoretically and empirically supported approach to investigating mood for use in UK, Hungarian and Italian athletes.

References

Beedie (2005). It's the POMS, it Measures Mood – Doesn't it? International Society of Sport Psychology (ISSP). *11th World Congress of Sport Psychology,* 15-19 August 2005, Sydney Convention and Exhibition Centre, Sydney, Australia.

Bentler, P. M. (1990). Comparative fit indices in structural models. *Psychological Bulletin, 107*, 238-246.

Bentler, P.M. (1995). *EQS structural equation program manual.* Encino, CA: Multivariate Software.

Bentler, P.M. and Wu, E.J.C. (1995). *EQS/Windows user's guide.* Encino, CA: Multivariate Software.

Browne, M. W., and Cudeck, R. (1993). Alternative ways of assessing model fit. In Bollen, K. A., and Long, J. S. (Eds.), *Testing structural equation models*, (pp.132-162). Newbury, CA: Sage.

Byrne, B.M. (1998). *Structural equation modelling with LISREL, PRELIS, and SIMPLIS: Basic concepts, applications and programming.* Mahwah, NJ: Lawrence Erlbaum.

Byrne, B.M. (2000). *Structural equation modelling with AMOS: Basic concepts, applications and programming.* Mahwah, NJ: Lawrence Erlbaum.

Grove, W.R., and Prapavessis, H. (1992) Preliminary evidence for the reliability and validity of an abbreviated Profile of Mood States. *International Journal of Sport Psychology, 23*, 93-109.

Hanin, Y. (2000). *Emotions in sport.* Champaign, IL: Human Kinetics.

Hewston, R., Lane, A. M., Karageorghis, C., and Nevill, A. M. (2005). The relationship between music, mood-regulation and coping style. *Journal of Sports Sciences, 22*, 175-176.

Hoyle, R. H., and Panter, A. T. (1995). Writing about structural equation models. In Hoyle, R. H. (Ed.), *Structural equation modeling: Concepts, issues, and applications*, (pp. 158-175). Newbury, CA: Sage.

Hu, L., and Bentler, P. M. (1999). Cutoff criteria for fit indexes in covariance structure analysis: Conventional criteria versus new alternatives. *Structural equation modelling, 6,* 1-55.

Jones, M. V., Lane, A. M., Bray, S. R., Uphill, M., and Catlin, J. (2005). Development of the Sport Emotions Questionnaire. *Journal of Sport and Exercise Psychology, 27*, 407-431.

Kline, P. (1998). *Handbook of psychological testing*. London: Routledge.

Lane, A. M. (2004). Measures of emotions and coping in sport. *In Coping and Emotion in Sport*. Pp255-271. Editors Lavallee, D., Thatcher, J., and Jones, M. Nova Science, NY.

Lane, A. M., and Jarrett, H. (2005). Mood changes following golf among senior recreational players. *Journal of Sports Science and Medicine, 4*, 47-51.

Lane, A. M., and Terry, P. C. (2000). The nature of mood: Development of a conceptual model with a focus on depression. *Journal of Applied Sport Psychology, 12*, 16-33.

Lane, H, J., Lane, A. M., and Matheson, H. (2004). Validity of the eating attitude test among exercisers. *Journal of Sports Science and Medicine, 3,* 244-253.

Matthews, G., Jones, D. M., and Chamberlain, A. G. (1990). Refining the measurement of mood: The UWIST Mood Adjective Checklist. *British Journal of Psychology, 81,* 17-42.

McNair, D. M., Lorr, M., and Droppleman, L. F. (1971). Manual for the Profile of Mood States. San Diego, CA: Educational and Industrial Testing Services.

McNair, D. M., Lorr, M., and Droppleman, L. F. (1992). Revised Manual for the Profile of Mood States. SanDiego, CA: Educational and Industrial Testing Services.

Schutz, R. W. (1994). Methodological issues and measurement problems in sport psychology. In S. Serpa, J. Alves, J., and V. Pataco (Eds.), *International Perspectives on Sport and Exercise Psychology*. (pp. 35-57). Morgantown, Fitness Information Technnology, Inc.

Soos, I., Lane, A. M., Leibinger, E., Karsai, I., and Hamar, P. (2005). Validity of the Profile of Mood States (SF) among Hungarian students. International Society of Sport Psychology (ISSP) 11th World Congress of Sport Psychology, 15-19 August 2005, Sydney Convention and Exhibition Centre, Sydney, Australia.

Soos, I., Leibinger, I., Karsai, I., and Hamar, P. (in press). Mood differences in university students in two countries. *Journal of Hospitality, Sport, Tourism, Leisure, Education.*

Speilberger, C. D. (1991). *Manual for the State-trait anger expression inventory*. Odessa, FL: Psychological Assessment Resources.

Steiger, J.H. (1990). Structural model evaluation and modification: An interval estimation approach. *Multivariate Behavioral Research,* 25, 173-180.

Terry, P. C., Lane, A. M., and Fogarty, G. (2003). Construct validity of the Profile of Mood States-A for use with adults. *Psychology of Sport and Exercise*, *4*, 125-139.

Terry, P. C., Lane, A. M., Lane, H. J., and Keohane, L. (1999). Development and validation of a mood measure for adolescents: POMS-A. *Journal of Sports Sciences, 17*, 861-872.

Tucker, L. R., and Lewis, C. (1973). A reliability coefficient for maximum likelihood factor analysis. *Psychometrika, 38*, 1-10.

Watson, D., Clark, L. A., and Tellegen, A. (1988). Development and validation of brief measures of positive and negative affect: The PANAS scales. *Journal of Personality and Social Psychology, 54*, 1063-1070.

In: Hot Topics in Sports and Athletics
Editor: Samuel R. Bakere, pp. 129-142

ISBN 978-1-60456-077-0

Chapter 8

Circadian Rhythms and Physical Activity

Sebastien Racinais
ASPETAR, Qatar Orthopedic and Sports Medicine Hospital,
Exercise and Sports Science Department, Doha, Qatar

Abstract

In a neutral and controlled environment, physical performance during a short-duration exercise fluctuates during the day with an acrophase close to 18:00 h. The diurnal increase in muscle power is mainly attributed to a diurnal increase in muscle force. This diurnal increase in muscle force is mainly attributed to a diurnal increase in muscle contractile properties. Today, the physiological basis of this variation in muscle contractile function remains unclear and represents a challenging topic in the future because the circadian variation in muscle force is generally in phase with the circadian variation in body core temperature. It is hypothesized that the diurnal increase in core temperature could have a beneficial passive warm-up effect.

It is possible to shift the acrophase of the muscle power variation by a couple of hours following a few days by adapting sleep and meal schedules. Moreover, the use of another source of passive warm-up (e.g., a warm environment) seems to blunt the diurnal variation in muscle power. With long duration exercise, the thermal stress induced by physical exercise in a warm (and humid) environment should be higher in the evening, when the initial body temperatures are the highest.

Physical activities have to be considered for their effect on health. For example, cardiac events occur mainly between 06:00 - 12:00 h and a vigorous physical activity could be a trigger for them. Clinicians should advise at risk patients to avoid exercise at this time-of-day. Physical activity can also have some beneficial effects. For example, physical activity increases the amplitude of some circadian variations in elderly people allowing for the improvement both nocturnal sleep quality (i.e., less) and diurnal vigilance.

Introduction

The biological rhythms may influence the physical abilities, however participation in regular physical activity may influence the biological rhythms. The first part of this chapter will focus on the diurnal variation in physical attributes. Firstly, the effect of circadian rhythm upon different physical abilities will be discussed. However, because most physical activities are performed during day-time, and thus low nocturnal values have only a poor functional significance, the second part of this chapter will focus on the effect of time-of-day upon physical performance (i.e., morning versus afternoon). Thirdly, how to control the diurnal variation in physical ability will be discussed. The effect of body temperature and its diurnal variations on the exercising body will be emphased.

From a broader point of view, the influence of circadian rhythms constitutes a challenging issue in medicine. For example, for several decades it has been known that the time-of-day at which chemotherapy administrated influences relapse rates in children (e.g. Rivard *et al.* 1985). In parallel, physical activity is also generally considered to induce chronic adaptation that reduces risk factors for many medical conditions (long term). Consequently, the second part of this chapter aims to link the triptych circadian rhythms, health, and physical activity by relating the effects of physical activity on health in regard to the circadian rhythms. Three examples will be used to highlight this complex relationship. In the first example, the well-known circadian rhythm in body core temperature will be considered for its consequences on thermoregulation and health during exercise. The diurnal increase in core temperature generally observed at rest persists during physical exercise (Reilly *et al.* 1984, Reilly et Brooks 1990). The thermal stress induced by a physical exercise should be higher in the evening, when the initial body temperatures are the highest (Reilly et Garret 1998). This could be particularly important for exercising in warm and humid environments where sweating fails to compensate for the increase in body temperature increase or for a patient with spinal cord injuries, with a loss or reduction in the ability to dissipate heat from below the level of lesion. In the second example, physical exercise will be considered as a risk factor for a cardiac event (Siscovick *et al.* 1984, Giri *et al.* 1999). This will be discussed in relation to the diurnal variation in the occurrence of cardiac events (Muller *et al.* 1987, Willich *et al.* 1989). In the third example, physical activity will be considered as a zeitgeber helping to maintain the circadian sleep-wake cycle in the elderly as temperature variations of the circadian rhythm are reduced with aging (Atkinson *et al.* 1992). This decrease is associated with an alteration of the sleep-wake cycle (Flamer 1996, Vitiello *et al.* 1997). Regular physical activity, however, can induce chronic adaptations in the amplitude of circadian rhythms (Atkinson *et al.* 1993). An improvement in the sleep-wake cycle (i.e. with better daytime vigilance and less wake-up time overnight) has been seen in the elderly subjects after a physical training program (Mauvieux *et al.* 2003).

I. Diurnal Variations in Physical Ability

I.1. Physical Ability and Circadian Rhythms

The ability to perform in middle- and long-duration events is generally considered to be linked to the athlete's maximal oxygen consumption; however, the circadian rhythm of this parameter remains unclear. Some of the studies have concluded that maximal oxygen consumption does not significantly fluctuate during the day (Faria and Drummond 1982, Reilly and Brooks 1982 and 1990, Jones and Hill 1995), whereas others have observed diurnal variation (Hill *et al.* 1988 and 1989b, Williams and Hill 1995) with, in some instances, no signiticant diurnal variation in performance itself (e.g. time to exhaustion) (Hill *et al.* 1988).

In short duration performances, the data is unequivocal and displays a diurnal fluctuation. Recent research supports and explains the observation of Rodahl (1976) that high-level swimmer perform better in the evening than in the morning. A significant circadian variation in both back and leg force, with an acrophase of the circadian rhythm at 16:53 h and 18:20 h, respectively, (Coldwells *et al.* 1994) has been observed. Futhermore, the peak torque produced by elbow flexors confirms these observations by displaying a circadian rhythm peaking at 17:30 (Gauthier *et al.* 1996).

Additionally, this circadian variation in muscle force (i.e., a value obtained in a laboratory during an isolated isometric contraction) seems to lead to a circadian variation in performance (e.g., a time, a distance, a length...). Performances recorded during an isolated movement (maximal jump) have previously been recorded to display a circadian variation with an acrophase close to 17:45 h (Reilly and Down 1986 and 1992). A similar variation was also observed for an anaerobic test (test of Margaria) with a calculated acrophase at 17:26 h (Reilly and Down 1992).

In controlled conditions, most studies have observed an acrophase in performance during short-duration exercise close to 18:00 h. Furthermore, the circadian variation in this kind of performance is generally in phase with the circadian variation in body core temperature (Reilly and Down 1986, 1992). Several studies have suggested that the simultaneous increases in core temperature (from oral or rectal data) and muscular power are causally related because the diurnal increase in core temperature may have a beneficial passive warm-up effect (Bernard *et al.* 1998, Melhim 1993, Racinais *et al.* 2004 and 2005a). However, the fact that the circadian rhythms in both body temperature and short-duration performance, are in phase doesn't represent evidence of causal link. This question remains unclear. The next objective in these research topics is to investigate the existence of a circadian variation in muscle temperature.

I.2. Physical Ability and Time-of-Day

We saw in the preceding paragraph that most of the studies concluded a circadian variation of the muscle force, and thus of the performance, during a short-duration exercise. However, the statistical significance of this circadian rhythm could be linked to low values during night whereas most of the physical activities (sport events, leisure or work) are performed during the day. A functional approach of the diurnal variation in physical abilities could be to investigate the existence of fluctuation during day-time rather than nocturnal nadir. In the literature, studies on the whole solar cycle (i.e., 24 h) generally use the terminology of 'circadian rhythms' whereas studies focusing on the day-time use 'time-of-day'.

From this point of view, it is relevant to highlight that most of the studies observed an improvement in performance during short-duration exercise during the day. For example, better performance were observed in the afternoon than in the morning for: vertical jump height (Bernard *et al.* 1998, Racinais *et al.* 2004), sprint running velocity (Javiere *et al.* 1996), maximal cycling power output (Bernard *et al.* 1998, Racinais *et al.* 2005b), or total work during 30 seconds (Melhim 1993) and 60 seconds (Hill *et al.* 1992) cycle exercise.

This diurnal fluctuation in muscle power can be a consequence of a modification in neural drive and/or a modification in muscle contractile function. The later seems to be the dominant factor. Skeletal muscle contractility is significantly greater in the afternoon than in the morning (Gauthier *et al.* 1996, Martin *et al.* 1999, Racinais *et al.* 2005a), whereas this is not the case for the muscle electrical activity (Gauthier *et al.* 1996, Racinais *et al.* 2005a). Racinais *et al.* (2005a) observed a large (+12%) increase in isometric force of the knee extensors during the day despite a decrease in muscle electrical activity. Similar data were previously observed by Gauthier *et al.* (1996) leading them to conclude that the vulnerability of the organism could be reduced by having the acrophase of different physiological parameters at different times. From a general point of view, muscle electrical activity is higher in the morning suggesting that the body may well have a protective mechanism that partially compensates for the diurnal variation in the muscle contractile properties by an opposite variation in the central command (Gauthier *et al.* 1996, Racinais *et al.* 2005a).

Thus, in summary, the diurnal increase in muscle power is mainly attributed to a diurnal increase in muscle force (Racinais *et al.* 2005b). This diurnal increase in muscle force is mainly attributed to a diurnal increase in muscle contractile properties (Gauthier *et al.* 1996, Martin *et al.* 1999, Racinais *et al.* 2005a). However, the physiological basis of this variation in muscle contractile function remained unclear and will represent a challenging topic in the future.

One proposed theory is that the circadian rhythm in body temperature could act as a passive warm-up for increasing muscle contractility (Racinais *et al.* 2005a), suggests that the low morning temperatures do not match the optimal conditions for muscle efficiency. This theory is partly based on the previous observation of a greater Ca^{2+} retention by the sarcoplasmic reticulum with a decrease in muscle temperature (Segal *et al.* 1986, Stein *et al.* 1982). If we explain the variation in muscle contractility by a variation in calcium concentration in the muscle fiber , this would not influence the muscle contractility during sub-maximal contractions, when the needs are lower. In line with this hypothesis, it is relevant to note that muscle contractility is significantly higher in the afternoon than in the morning during high intensity contractions (i.e., from 75% to 100% of max), but not during contractions at 25% or 50% of max (Racinais *et al.* 2005a). However, Martin *et al.* (1999) advanced the hypothesis that these mechanisms were not only muscle temperature-dependent, but also controlled by the daytime hormonal fluctuations. Furthermore, it is generally considered that it is local temperature of the exercising limbs rather than core temperature which influences maximal muscle power (Falk *et al.* 1998), but the diurnal fluctuation in muscle temperature was never investigated yet. Thus, today, we can only conclude that there is currently insufficient data available to explain with certitude the cause of the variation in muscle contractile state as a function of time-of-day.

I.3. How to Control the Diurnal Variation in Physical Ability

The previous paragraph presented the diurnal variation in some physical abilities. But, if it is very useful to know and understand these fluctuations, athletes and coaches need also to know how to control them. The best and easiest way to obtain the best performance possible is to schedule the recording at the time-of-day corresponding to the acrophase of the athlete for this performance. However, this solution may be not possible, especially in official events. So, if the time of the event can not be adapted to the athlete, the athlete has to adapt himself to the time of the event. In this paragraph, we will see that this kind of adaptation is possible.

The first possibility existing for an athlete to have a small shift in his circadian rhythm is to have a shift in his zeitgebers. Generally, it is impossible to change the night-day cycle. However, if the alternation in light and dark are the main zeitgeber for most of the animals, the social activities are a major zeitgeber in humans. A very interesting study was performed by Javierre *et al.* (1996) with national level sprinters. In this experiment, they recorded the diurnal fluctuations in 80 m sprint performance after different modifications in sleep and/or meal schedules. Their data showed that to postpone both meal and sleep schedules by 2 hours shifts the initial fluctuation in performance by two hours later. Inversely, to advance both meal and sleep schedules by two hours lead a shift of the initial fluctuation in performance by two hours earlier. In summary, two points particularly relevant in their results: (i) it is possible to have a shift the acrophase of your performance in a task in which you specialise, and (ii) this shift was obtained within only two days (Javierre *et al.* 1996).

It is also possible to influence the natural diurnal fluctuation in performance by regularly practicing a physical activity at a given time-of-day. Indeed, muscle power seems to progress after training specifically with time-of-day of training (Souissi *et al.* 2002). Likewise, a greater improvement in aerobic performances seems also to occur at the time-of-day at which training was regularly performed (Hill *et al.* 1989a, 1998). A short-term adaptation to the time-of-day for exercising has also been emphasized from one day to the following day (Edwards *et al.* 2005).

While controlling sleep, meal and exercise schedules modifies or to shifts the diurnal variation in performance, some other conditions can completely blunt this diurnal fluctuation. This is especially the case of a warm environment. As detailed above, in temperate conditions, short-duration performance is generally increased by the end of the afternoon, at the peak of the core temperature curve (Coldwells *et al.* 1994, Melhim 1993, Reilly and Down 1986, 1992, Bernard *et al.* 1998, Deschenes *et al.* 1998). Even if the circadian rhythm in core temperature is not necessarily the cause of the rhythm in muscle performance, some studies have suggested that the simultaneous increases in both body temperature and muscle power are causally related (Coldwells *et al.* 1994, Melhim 1993, Bernard *et al.* 1998, Racinais *et al.* 2004a,b, 2005a). These studies based their hypothesis on previous work showing that an increase in muscle temperature could increase muscle power (i.e. Bergh and Ekblom 1979) and considered the diurnal increase in body temperature as a passive warm-up (Bernard *et al.* 1998, Melhim 1993, Racinais *et al.* 2004a,b) increasing muscle contractility (Racinais *et al.* 2005a).

In parallel with the diurnal variation in body temperature, a variation in environmental temperature can influence muscle power. A moderately hot environment has been shown to enhance jump performance (Hue *et al.* 2003) and cycle power (Falk *et al.* 1998). These observations are confirmed by a lot of studies showing that a local passive warm-up increased muscle performance (e.g., Bergh and Ekblom 1979, Bergh 1980, Davies and Young 1985, Sargeant 1987, Crowley *et al.* 1991). In summary, time-of-day (i.e., the diurnal increase in body temperature) and a warm environment seems to represent two factors increasing muscle performance by a passive warm-up effect. So, the question is to know whether an external passive warm-up controls the passive warm-up effect of the time-of-day. In line with this hypothesis, a study conducted in a tropical environment failed to show any circadian variation in muscle power, suggesting that the hot and humid environment (28.1°C and 63% of relative humidity) may have blunted the circadian rhythm in muscular power (Racinais *et al.* 2004a). This study raised intriguing questions about the cause of this stability. Two suggestions seemed reasonable: (i) a long-term adaptation to the environmental conditions or (ii) an instantaneous effect of the testing conditions. Some recent studies comparing diurnal variation (i.e., morning versus afternoon) in muscle power in the same subject in function of the environmental temperature observed an interaction effect within time-of-day and environmental conditions (Racinais *et al.* 2004b, 2005a), showing that it was the testing condition that blunted the diurnal variation in muscle power. Interestingly, a warm environment only facilitates improved muscle power (Racinais *et al.* 2004b) and contractility (2005a) in the morning, when body temperature is at its lowest. These findings suggest that these two passive warm-up effects have no additional effect on the improvement in muscle power and there is possibly a threshold for passive warm-up effects, above which additional sources of warm-up have no additional effect. (Racinais *et al.* 2006). In summary, athletes and coaches maybe able to blunt the diurnal variation in muscle power by using another source of passive warm-up (Racinais *et al.* 2004, 2005, and 2006).

II. Circadian Variation in Physical Ability: Effect on Health

II.1. Physical Activity and Circadian Variation in Temperature

One of the most known circadian rhythms is core temperature. Human core temperature is generally measured by rectally and displays an acrophase in the late afternoon, close to 18:00 h (Waterhouse *et al.* 1993). This circadian rhythm is mainly endogenous and persists in free-living conditions, without influence of the zeitgebers (Colin *et al.* 1968). Even if the absolute recorded values are dependent of the methodology (i.e., different depth of insertion within a probe and a clinical thermometer), it is well established that rectal temperature displays a diurnal increase whether measured by a rectal probe (Bernard *et al.* 1998, Racinais *et al.* 2005b) or clinical thermometer (Atkinson *et al.* 1993, Racinais *et al.* 2004, 2005a).

Circadian variations in body temperature are considered to lead many of other circadian variations but can have its own consequences on health, especially during exercise. During exercise, muscle contraction produces heat leading to a proportional relation within relative work intensity and core temperature (Saltin *et al.* 1968). For example, during moderate exercise, muscle temperature increases quickly from a basal value close to 35°C, rising above rectal temperature within 3 to 5 min before plateauing after 10 to 20 minutes. In a neutral environment, core temperature increases when muscle temperature becomes higher than rectal temperature but different thermoregulatory systems attempt to preserve homeostasis. During prolonged exercise the majority of heat dissipation is facilitated by evaporation, while convection, conduction, and radiation play are smaller role. A part of the heat is also stored in the body leading to an increase in core temperature. However, the storage possibilities are limited and more and more studies state core -and may be cerebral- temperature as the limiting factor of aerobic performance in warm environment (Caputa *et al.* 1986, Brück and Olschewski 1987, Gonzales-Alonzo *et al.* 1999). For trained subjects, cessation of activity in warm environment seems to occur at a given critical core temperature whatever the exercise intensity, the heat storage capacity, the acclimatizing state, the initial temperature or the skin temperature (Brück and Olshewski 1987, Gonzales-Alonso *et al.* 1999). Accordingly, rats stop exercising in hot environment at the same abdominal and cerebral temperature whatever the modification made to their initial temperature (Fuller *et al.* 1998, Walters *et al.* 2000). Furthermore, if the cerebral temperature of a goat is increased close to 42°C by a local warm-up, they reduced their velocity or refuse to move (Caputa *et al.* 1986).

In human body, from a basal temperature close to 37°C to a limit close to 40°C (Gonzales-Alonso *et al.* 1999), the heat storages possibilities seem inadequate. From this point of view, the natural circadian variation in core temperature seems to be an important point to consider. Indeed, an increase in body temperature before a long-duration exercise can decrease performance by altering the heat storage capacity (Nadel 1987, Gonzales-Alonso *et al.* 1999). Similarly, pre-cooling can increase the heat storage capacity and increase the running time to exhaustion (Lee and Haymes 1995, Gonzales-Alonso *et al.* 1999). Thus, we can hypothesis that the circadian variation in core temperature will modify the heat storage capacity and thus the ability to exercise. This hypothesis is valid only when heat dissipation fails to maintained homeostasis and thus the heat storage capacity becomes a limiting factor. This is notably the case in warm and humid environment, when required evaporative cooling exceeds the evaporative capacity of the environment (Shapiro *et al.* 1998). The diurnal variation in core temperature persisting during physical exercise (Reilly *et al.* 1984, Reilly and Brooks 1990) and the thermal stress induced by physical exercise in warm (and humid) environment should be higher in the evening, when the initial body temperatures are at its highest (Reilly and Garret 1998). However, this could auto regulated by the human body. Indeed, it seems that the increase in body temperature during prolonged exercise could be greater in the morning, leading to a reduction in the amplitude of the circadian variation as exercise progress (Aldemir *et al.* 2000).

Thus, this topic needs further research in warm environments is required to investigate the effect the circadian rhythm in core temperature on thermoregulation capacity during exercise. An additional source of thermoregulation limitation should also be investigated in regard to the circadian rhythm in core temperature in patients with spinal cord injuries can suffer from a reduction or loss in ability to dissipate heat from below the level of lesion.

II.2. Physical Activity and Circadian Variations in Cardiac Event

From a chronobiological point of view, the rate of occurrence in cardiac events seems to display circadian variations. Muller *et al.* (1987) observed a prominent circadian variation of sudden cardiac death, with a low incidence during the night and an increased incidence from 07:00 to 11:00. a.m. These data are confirmed by the observation of Willich *et al.* (1989) that the incidence of myocardial infarction was markedly increased between 06:00 and 12:00 a.m. compared with other times of day. The amplitude of variation is relatively important as myocardial infarction occurred 3.8 times more frequently between 08:00 and 09:00 (hour of maximum incidence) than between 00:00 and 01:00 a.m. (hour of minimum incidence) (Willich *et al.* 1989). However, these differences are also linked to the different levels of activity and to the stress involved with the wake-up itself (Atkinson *et al.* 2006).

Moreover, vigorous physical activity acutely increases the risk of sudden cardiac death (Siscovick *et al.* 1984)http://circ.ahajournals.org/cgi/content/full/107/24/3109 - R57-130157# R57-130157 and myocardial infarction (Giri *et al.* 1999)http://circ.ahajournals.org/cgi/ content/full/107/24/3109 - R59-130157#R59-130157 among individuals with both diagnosed and occult heart disease. Thus, because acute cardiac events occur mainly between 06:00 - 12:00 a.m. and that physical activity is generally thought to be a trigger for such events, clinicians should advise patients already at risk not to exercise in the morning. However many people prefer this time-of-day for recreational activities and household chores, while the general preference of middle-aged and elderly people scheduling activity and sleep at earlier times than young adults (Atkinson *et al.* 2006).

It is important to know how to make morning recreational activities safe. At this point, it is particularly relevant to consider that supervised exercise programs seem to be safe for cardiac patients, irrespective of time-of-day (Atkinson *et al.* 2006), while the incidence of cardiac events is low in coronary artery disease patients during regular, sub-maximal exercise whether performed in the morning or afternoon (Murray *et al.* 1993). Moreover, from a general point of view, regular sub-maximal exercises are generally considered to be beneficial for health. Regular physical activity using large muscle groups, such as walking, running, or swimming, produces cardiovascular adaptations that increase exercise capacity, endurance, and skeletal muscle strength. Habitual physical activity also prevents the development of coronary artery disease and reduces symptoms in patients with established cardiovascular disease (Statement from the Council on Clinical Cardiology and Council on Nutrition, Physical Activity, and Metabolism, 2003). But, if exercise programs for cardiac patients have generally a 2- to 6-months supervised period of sub-maximal exercise, they are generally followed by unsupervised activity in the subsequent months (Atkinson *et al.* 2006).

Consequently, the question can be reformulated to know if the supervised exercise program can reduce the risk of a cardiac event if the patients exercise in the morning thereafter.

In this way, it is particularly relevant to consider than physical training can induce some adaptation specific to the time-of-day in which the training is performed. For example, as presented in the first section of this chapter, a greater improvement in aerobic performances seems to occur at the time-of-day at which training was regularly performed (Hill *et al.* 1989a, 1998). It may be useful for physicians to introduce supervised sub-maximal exercise in the morning during the supervised program. That could induce specific adaptations to reduce the risk of cardiac event in the subsequent physical activity, if, against medical advice, the patients perform strenuous activity in the morning.

II.3. Physical Activity and Circadian Rhythm in Elderly

On other important relation within biological rhythms, physical exercise and health concerns the beneficial effects of physical training. Chronic physical activity is considered to have beneficial effect in ederly on both physiological (e.g., the risk of cardiovascular event, Andrawes *et al.* 2005) and cognitive (Renaud and Bherer 2005) aging, but physical activity can also act as a zeitgeber. This point is particularly relevant in this population displaying a loss of the stability of their circadian rhythm.

Indeed, some circadian variations are blunted with aging (e.g., mood state, Atkinson *et al.* 1992) and others persist but with a reduction in amplitude (e.g., core temperature, Atkinson *et al.* 1992). In addition to the reduction in the amplitude of the circadian rhythms, an earlier acrophase is also observed in elderly (Atkinson *et al.* 1992). Moreover, aging leads an alteration of the sleep-wake rhythm with nap period during the day and a loss in quality/continuity of the nocturnal sleep (Flamer 1996, Vitiello *et al.* 1997).

However, regular physical activity induces chronic adaptations such as an increase in circadian variations amplitude in young subjects (Atkinson *et al.* 1993). The question is to know whether maintaining physical activity throughout the aging process can maintain the standard sleep-wake cycle. The beneficial effect of physical activity for better aging is well documented (for a review, see the position stand of the American College of Sports Medicine 1998). But the problem is that, in parallel of alterations in biological rhythm, physical activity generally decreases with aging in relation to a more sedentary lifestyle and/or a loss in mobility.

Concerning the biological rhythms, Mauvieux *et al.* (2003) observed a significant increase in the amplitude of the circadian rhythm in core temperature after four months of training. From a theoretical point of view, this observation confirms in an elderly population the observation of Atkinson *et al.* (1993) in young subjects. From a functional point of view, this increases in the amplitude of the circadian variation in core temperature was associated to an improvement in both nocturnal sleep quality (i.e., less wake-up) and diurnal vigilance (Mauvieux *et al.* 2003). It seems important to highlight that, despite some physiological adaptation to training persist for a long time, the zeitgeber action of the physical activity does not. Regular physical activity is needed to help maintain both the sleep-wake cycle and sleep quality. It is also interesting to consider that it is the increase in core temperature during exercise which could lead amelioration in sleep quality (Horne and Staff 1983). Indeed, a passive or active increase in core temperature allows for an increase in the slow-wave sleep in the subsequent night and thus improves the sleep-wake cycle (Horne et Staff 1983, Horne 1992).

Conclusion

In summary, the relationship between circadian rhythms and physical activity is complex and bidirectional. On one hand, biological rhythms influence physical abilities during short-duration exercise. This influence seems to be lead by a diurnal variation in muscle contractile properties, which may be related with the circadian rhythm in core temperature. On the other hand, physical activity can also influence the biological rhythms. This influence can allow modification in the amplitude of a rhythm (i.e., an active life generally leads to an increase in amplitude) or its synchronization in regard to the solar day (i.e., possibility to shift the acrophase by a few hours or to stabilize a rhythm). In this chapter, we tried to highlight some possible ways for future research. In view of the importance given to the circadian rhythm in core temperature and for the synchronization of the other rhythms, we think that the possibility of a diurnal variation in muscle temperature should be investigated. Indeed, it is generally considered that it is local temperature of the exercising muscle rather than core temperature that influences muscle power.

Future research should also continue to investigate the adaptation in patient, worker and athletes under the influence of perturbations of their endogenous circadian rhythms. The perturbations generally analyzed are notably shift work or jet lag but another source of perturbation should be investigated in athletes in the following years. During the holy month of Ramadan Muslims all over the world fast everyday for 4 weeks between the hours of sunrise to sunset. This special pattern of alimentation represents a perturbation of the habitual rhythm of life. Based on the 10 month lunar calendar Ramadan starts 10 days earlier each year, which could possibly impact on Muslim athletes yearly training and competition cycles (Grantham *et al.* 2006).

References

[1] Aldemir H, Atkinson G, Cable T, Edwards B, Waterhouse J, Reilly T. (2000). A comparison of the immediate effects of moderate exercise in the early morning and late afternoon on core temperature and cutaneous thermoregulatory mechanisms. *Chronobiol. Int.* 17: 197-207.

[2] American College of Sports Medicine. (1998). ACSM position stand on exercise and physical activity for older adults. *Med. Sci. Sports Exerc.* 30: 992-1008.

[3] Andrawes WF, Bussy C, Belmin J. (2005). Prevention of cardiovascular events in elderly people. *Drugs Aging.* 22: 859-876.

[4] Atkinson G, Coldwells A, Reilly T, Waterhouse J. (1992). Effects of age on circadian rhythms in physical performance and mood states. *J. Interdisciplin. Cycle Res.* 23: 186-188.

[5] Atkinson G, Coldwells A, Reilly T, Waterhouse J. (1993). A comparison of circadian rhythms in work performance between physical active and inactive subjects. *Ergonomics.* 16: 273-281.

[6] Atkinson G, Drust B, George K, Reilly T, Waterhouse J. (2006). Chronobiological considerations for exercise and heart disease. *Sports Med.* 36: 487-500.

[7] Bergh U, Ekblom B. (1979). Influence of muscle temperature on maximal muscle strength and power output in human skeletal muscles. *Acta Physiol. Scand.* 107: 33-37.

[8] Bergh U. (1980). Human power at submaximal body temperature. *Acta Physiol. Scand.* Suppl: 478.

[9] Bernard T, Giacomoni M, Gavarry O, Seymat M, Falgairette G. (1998a). Time-of-day effects in maximal anaerobic leg exercise. *Eur. J. Appl. Physiol.* 77: 133-138.

[10]Bruck K, Olschewski H. (1987). Body temperature related factors diminishing the drive to exercise. *Can. J. Physiol. Pharmacol.* 65: 1274-1280.

[11]Caputa M, Feistkorn G, Jessen C. (1986). Effects of brain and trunk temperatures on exercise performance in goats. *Pflugers. Arch.* 406: 184–189.

[12]Coldwells A, Atkinson G, Reilly T. (1994). Sources of variation in back and leg dynamometry. *Ergonomics.* 37: 79-86.

[13]Colin J, Timbal J, Boutelier C, Houdas Y, Siffre M. (1968). Rhythm of the rectal temperature during a 6-month free-running experiment. *J. Appl. Physiol.* 25: 170-1 76.

[14]Council on Clinical Cardiology (Subcommittee on Exercise, Rehabilitation, and Prevention) and Council on Nutrition, Physical Activity, and Metabolism (Subcommittee on Physical Activity): Thompson PD, Buchner D, Piña IL, Balady GJ, Williams MA, Marcus BH, Berra K, Blair SN, Costa F, Franklin B, Fletcher GF, Gordon NF, Pate RR, Rodriguez BL, Yancey AK, Wenger NK. (2003). Exercise and Physical Activity in the Prevention and Treatment of Atherosclerotic Cardiovascular Disease. *Circulation.* 107: 3109.

[15]Crowley GC, Garg A, Lohn MS, Van Someren N, Wade AJ. (1991). Effects of cooling the legs on performance in a standard Wingate anaerobic test. *Br. J. Sports Med.* 25: 200-203.

[16]Davies CT, Young K. (1985). Effect of heating on the contractile properties of triceps surae and maximal power output during jumping in elderly men. *Gerontology.* 31: 1-5.

[17]Deschenes MR, Kraemer WJ, Bush JA, Doughty TA, Kim D, Mullen KM, Ramsey K. (1998). Biorhythmic influences on functional capacity of human muscle and physiological responses. *Med. Sci. Sports Exerc.* 30: 1399-1407.

[18]Edwards BJ, Edwards W, Waterhouse J, Atkinson G, Reilly T. (2005). Can Cycling Performance in an Early Morning, Laboratory-Based Cycle Time-Trial be Improved by Morning Exercise the Day Before? *Int. J. Sports Med.* 26: 651-656.

[19]Falk B, Radom-Isaac S, Hoffmann JR, Wang Y, Yarom Y, Magazanik A, Weinstein Y. (1998). The effect of heat exposure on performance of and recovery from high-intensity, intermittent exercise. *Int. J. Sports Med.* 19: 1-6.

[20]Faria IE, Drummond BJ. (1982). Circadian changes in resting heart rate and body temperature, maximal oxygen consumption and perceived exertion. *Ergonomics.* 25: 381-386.

[21]Flamer HE. (1996). Sleep disorders in the elderly. *Aust. N Z J. Med.* 26: 96-104.

[22]Fuller A, Carter RN, Mitchell D. (1998). Brain and abdominal temperatures at fatigue in rats exercising in the heat. *J. Appl. Physiol.* 84: 877–883.

[23]Gauthier A, Davenne D, Martin A, Cometti G, Van Hoecke J. (1996). Diurnal rhythm of the muscular performance of elbow flexors during isometric contractions. *Chronobiology International.* 13: 135-146.

[24]Giri S, Thompson PD, Kiernan FJ, Clive J, Fram DB, Mitchel JF, Hirst JA, McKay RG, Waters DD. (1999). Clinical and angiographic characteristics of exertion-related acute myocardial infarction. *JAMA.* 282: 1731–1736.

[25]Gonzalez-Alonso J, Teller C, Andersen SL, Jensen FB, Hyldig T, Nielsen B. (1999). Influence of body temperature on the development of fatigue during prolonged exercise in the heat. *J. Appl. Physiol.* 86: 1032–1039.

[26]Grantham JR, Belhaj J, O'Brien B, Balasekaran G. (2006). The effect of 4 weeks fasting during Ramadan upon isokinetic knee flexor/extensor performance. *Med. Sci. Sports Exerc.* 38: S337.

[27]Hill DW, Borden DO, Darnaby KM, Hendricks DN, Hill CM. (1992). Effect of time of day on aerobic and anaerobic responses to high-intensity exercise. *Can. J. Sport Sci.* 17: 316-319.

[28]Hill DW, Cureton KJ, Collins MA, Grisham SC. (1988). Diurnal variations in responses to exercise of "morning types" and "evening types". *J. Sports Med.* 28: 213-219.

[29]Hill DW, Cureton KJ, Collins MA. (1989a). Circadian specificity in exercise training. *Ergonomics.* 32: 79-92.

[30]Hill DW, Cureton KJ, Collins MA. (1989b). Effect of time of day on perceived exertion at work rates above and below the ventilatory threshold. *R. Q. Exerc. Sports.* 60: 127-133.

[31]Hill DW, Leiferman JA, Lynch NA, Dangelmaier BS, Burt SE. (1998). Temporal specificity in adaptations to high-intensity exercise training. *Med. Sci. Sports Exerc.* 30. 450-455.

[32]Horne J, Staff L. (1983). Exercise and sleep: body-heating effects. *Sleep.* 1: 36-46.

[33]Horne J. (1992). Human slow wave sleep: a review and appraisal of recent findings, with implications for sleep functions, and psychiatric illness. *Experientia.* 4: 941-954.

[34]Hue O, Coman F, Blonc S, Hertogh C. (2003). Effect of tropical climate on performance during repeated jump-and-reach tests. *J. Sports Med. Phys. Fitness.* 43: 475-480.

[35]Javierre C, Calvo M, Diez A, Garrido E, Segura R, Ventura JL. (1996). Influence of sleep and meal schedules on performance peaks in competitive sprinters. *Int. J. Sports Med.* 17: 404-408.

[36]Jones HA, Hill DW. (1995). responses to incremental and constant power exercise tests at different times of day. *Med. Sci. Sports Exerc.* 27: S109.

[37]Lee DT, Haymes EM. (1995). Exercise duration and thermoregulatory responses after whole body precooling. *J. Appl. Physiol.* 79: 1971-1976.

[38]Martin A, Carpentier A, Guissard N, Van Hoecke J, Duchateau J. (1999). Effect of time of day on force variation in a human muscle. *Muscle Nerve.* 22: 1380-1387.

[39]Mauvieux B, Davenne D, Gruau S, Sesboue B, Denise P. (2003). Physical training effect on the circadian rhythm of the temperature and the sleep-activity cycle in the elderly. *Science and Sports.* 18: 93-103.

[40]Melhim AF. (1993). Investigation of circadian rhythms in peak power and mean power of female physical education students. *Int. J. Sports Med.* 14: 303-306.

[41]Muller JE, Ludmer PL, Willich SN, Tofler GH, Aylmer G, Klangos I, Stone PH. (1987). Circadian variation in the frequency of sudden cardiac death. *Circulation.* 75:131-138.

[42]Murray PM, Herrington DM, Pettus CW, Miller HS, Cantwell JD, Little WC. (1993). Should patients with heart disease exercise in the morning or afternoon? *Arch. Intern. Med.* 153: 833-836.

[43]Nadel ER. (1987). Prolonged exercise and high and low ambient temperatures. *Can. J. Sport Sci.* 12: 140S-142S.

[44]Racinais S, Blonc S, Hue O. (2005b). Effects of active warm-up and diurnal increase in temperature on muscular power. *Med. Sci. Sports Exerc.* 37: 2134-2139.

[45]Racinais S, Blonc S, Jonville S, Hue O. (2005a). Time-of-day influences the environmental effects on muscle force and contractility. *Med. Sci. Sports Exerc.* 37: 256-261.

[46]Racinais S, Chamari K, Hachana Y, Bartagi Z, Blonc S, Hue O. (2006). Effect of an acute hot and dry exposure in moderately warm and humid environment on muscle performance at different time-of-day. *Int. J. Sports Med.* 27: 49-54.

[47]Racinais S, Hue O, Blonc S. (2004b). Time-of-day effects on anaerobic muscular power in a moderately warm environment. *Chronobiol. Int.* 21: 485-495.

[48]Racinais S, Hue O, Hertogh C, Damiani M, Blonc S. (2004a). Time-of-day effects in maximal anaerobic leg exercise in tropical environment: a first approach. *Int. J. Sports Med.* 25: 186-190.

[49]Reilly T, Brooks GA. (1982). Investigation of circadian rhythms in metabolic responses to exercise. *Ergonomics.* 25: 1093-1107.

[50]Reilly T, Brooks GA. (1990). Selective persistence of circadian rhythms in physiological responses to exercise. *Chronobiol. Int.* 7: 59-67.

[51]Reilly T, Down A. (1986). Circadian variation in the standing broad jump. *Perceptual and Motor Skills.* 62: 830.

[52]Reilly T, Down A. (1992). Investigation of circadian rhythms in anaerobic power and capacity of the legs. *J. Sports Med. Phys. Fitness.* 32: 343-347.

[53]Reilly T, Garret R (1998). Investigation of diurnal variation in sustained exercise performance. *Ergonomics.* 41: 1085-1094.

[54]Reilly T, Robinson G, Minors DS. (1984). Some circulatory responses to exercise at different times of day. *Med. Sci. Sports Exerc.* 16: 477-482.

[55]Renaud M, Bherer L. (2005). Impact on physical fitness on cognitive aging. *Psychol. Neuropsychiatr. Vieil.* 3: 199-206.

[56]Rodahl A, O'Brien M, Firth RG. (1976). Diurnal variation in performance of competitive swimmers. *J. Sports Med. Phys. Fitness.* 16: 72-76.

[57]Saltin B, Gagge AP, Stolwijk JA. (1968). Muscle temperature during submaximal exercise in man. *J. Appl. Physiol.* 25: 679-688.

[58]Sargeant AJ. (1987). Effect of muscle temperature on leg extension force and short-term power output in humans. *Eur. J. Appl. Physiol. Occup. Physiol.* 56: 693-698.

[59]Segal SS, Faulkner JA, White TP. (1986). Skeletal muscle fatigue in vitro is temperature dependent. *J. Appl. Physiol.* 61: 660-665.

[60]Shapiro Y, Moran D, Epstein Y. (1998). Acclimatization strategies – preparing for exercise in the heat. *Int. J. Sports Med.* 19: S161-S163.

[61]Siscovick DS, Weiss NS, Fletcher RH, Lasky T. (1984). The incidence of primary cardiac arrest during vigorous exercise. *N. Engl. J. Med.* 311: 874–877.

[62]Souissi N, Gauthier A, Sesboüé B, Larue J, Davenne D. (2002). Effects of regular training at the same time of day on diurnal fluctuations in muscular performance. *J. Sports Sci.* 20: 929-937.

[63]Stein RB, Gordon T, Shriver J. (1982). Temperature dependence of mammalian muscle contractions and ATPase activities. *Biophys. J.* 40: 97-107.

[64]Vitiello MV, Schwartz RS, Davis MW. (1997). Sleep disorders and aging: understanding the causes. *J. Gerontol. A Biol. Sci. Med. Sci.* 5: M189-191.

[65]Walters TJ, Ryan KL, Tate LM, Mason PA. (2000). Exercise in the heat is limited by a critical internal temperature. *J. Appl. Physiol.* 89: 799-806.

[66]Waterhouse JM, Minors DS, Folkard S. (1993). Estimating the endogenous component of the circadian rhythm of the rectal temperature in humans undergoing normal sleep/activity schedules. *J. Interdisciplin Cycle Res.* 24: 197-211.

[67]Williams CS, Hill DW. (1995). The effect of time of day on $\dot{V}O_2$ kinetics and $\dot{V}O_2$ max during high-intensity exercise. *Med. Sci. Sports Exerc.* 27: S109.

[68]Willich SN, Linderer T, Wegscheider K, Leizorovicz A, Alamercery I, Schroder R. (1989). Increased morning incidence of myocardial infarction in the ISAM Study: absence with prior beta-adrenergic blockade. ISAM Study Group. *Circulation.* 80: 853-858.

In: Hot Topics in Sports and Athletics
Editor: Samuel R. Bakere, pp. 143-157

ISBN 978-1-60456-077-0

Chapter 9

Coach and Athlete Burnout: The Role of Coaches' Decision-Making Style

Brandonn S. Harris and Andrew C. Ostrow
West Virginia University

Abstract

Recent burnout research has examined coaches and athletes collectively to determine the influence of coach behaviors on coach and athlete burnout. Results revealed a potential incongruity between decision-making behaviors and their influence on coach and athlete burnout. Therefore, the present study examined relationships between decision-making styles of coaches and burnout among coaches and athletes; gender influence on burnout was also examined. Collegiate swimmers and swimming coaches completed questionnaires assessing burnout and decision-making behaviors. Results revealed a significant relationship between athlete burnout and autocratic coaching behaviors. A significant inverse relationship emerged between athlete burnout and democratic behaviors. Significant main effects were found for democratic behaviors on exhaustion and depersonalization subscales; swimmers perceiving fewer democratic behaviors scored higher on these subscales. No significant relationships or gender differences were found with the coaches. Results suggest that coaches eliciting feedback from athletes could reduce the likelihood of burnout among those athletes without predisposing themselves.

Keywords: Coach and Athlete Burnout, Decision-Making, Leadership.

Burnout has become a topic of increasing interest to the sport community with some even suggesting that burnout has become synonymous with sports (Lai & Wiggins, 2003). When asked what feelings they associate with being burned out, athletes and coaches often cite internal and external sources of pressure, physical and mental exhaustion, mood changes, increased anxiety, and lack of caring (Weinberg & Gould, 2007). As both athletes and coaches experiencing burnout can end up mentally and physically withdrawing from a sport they once used to enjoy, it is apparent that a great deal of significance rests in understanding burnout.

With the coach and athlete populations having received research attention individually, recent studies have examined both groups collectively to determine the influence of coaching behaviors on coach and athlete burnout (Price & Weiss, 2000; Udry, Gould, Bridges, & Tuffey, 1997; Vealey, Armstrong, Comar, & Greenleaf, 1998). Related research on coaching behaviors has also noted that discrepancies between athletes' perceived and preferred leader/coach behaviors can contribute to dissatisfaction with athletes' sport experiences (Chelladurai, 1984). While this may be true, coach and athlete burnout may be another factor to consider that could result from this discrepancy. In noting that athletes cite severe practice conditions as the most important reason for their own burnout, Vealey et al. (1998) suggested the behaviors of coaches who are typically responsible for the practice conditions may be a critical component worthy of consideration in the occurrence of burnout among athletes. Although this premise guided their own research on athlete burnout, relatively little attention has been given to the effect coaches' behaviors, particularly decision-making styles, have on the occurrence of burnout in both coaches and athletes.

Research Regarding Decision-Making and Burnout in Sport

One relevant study to this line of research in the coaching population was conducted by Dale and Weinberg (1989). These authors studied leadership style and burnout in coaches and found those utilizing a consideration style evidenced greater emotional exhaustion and depersonalization, two common indicators of burnout. The authors suggested coaches with this style of leadership may become more emotionally involved with their teams, often giving more to their team than themselves. Price and Weiss (2000) found similar results in their research. Their study revealed that coaches reporting greater levels of burnout were perceived by their athletes to utilize democratic decision-making behaviors regarding their sport. However, in contrast to these two studies, Kelley, Eklund, and Ritter-Taylor (1999) found a democratic style of leadership to be associated with lower levels of burnout among coaches.

This line of burnout and leadership behavior research has also yielded some potentially troubling results, specifically the potential incongruity between decision-making styles and burnout among athletes and coaches that becomes apparent when examining the athlete burnout and leadership research. Vealey et al. (1998) examined the influence of perceived coaching behaviors on athlete burnout. Results indicated that athletes who scored higher on a burnout inventory also perceived their coach's leadership style to be more autocratic in nature. Price and Weiss (2000) also found that athletes reported higher levels of burnout in response to perceived autocratic coaching behaviors and less burnout in response to a democratic style of decision-making.

Collectively, these studies suggest that a decision-making style of coaches that has been linked to higher levels of burnout in coaches (democratic) is one that may aid in protecting athletes from experiencing burnout. Further, a decision-making style of coaches that has been correlated with higher levels of burnout in athletes (autocratic) is one that might reduce the likelihood of coaches experiencing burnout.

Research Regarding Gender and Burnout in Sport

In addition to leadership influences on coach and athlete burnout, research has examined the role gender plays in coach burnout; however, equivocal findings have been found (Davenport, 1998). Caccese and Mayerberg (1984) administered the Maslach Burnout Inventory (Maslach & Jackson, 1981) to 231 collegiate head coaches. Their results indicated that female coaches experienced significantly higher levels of burnout denoted by greater levels of emotional exhaustion and lower levels of personal accomplishments than their counterparts. No gender differences were found regarding the depersonalization subscale. Results have been mirrored by other studies regarding the emotional exhaustion subscale (Kelley, 1994; Kelley, et al., 1999; Pastore & Judd, 1993; Vealey, Udry, Zimmerman, & Soliday, 1992). However, Pastore and Judd (1993) and Vealey and colleagues (1992) were unable to demonstrate any gender differences regarding the personal accomplishment subscale. While many of these studies have found no gender differences regarding the depersonalization subscale of the MBI, others have suggested males experience greater levels of depersonalization than females (Dale & Weinberg, 1989). It can be concluded that gender differences in burnout among coaches needs further examination to help clarify the inconsistent findings of the previous research.

Interestingly, gender differences in burnout among athletes have received little research attention. Lai and Wiggins (2003) examined burnout perceptions in collegiate soccer players. Their hypotheses were formulated based on gender and burnout research conducted with coaches. They found that while burnout symptoms significantly increased over the course of a competitive season, no gender differences in burnout perceptions were present. The authors suggested that future research address possible gender differences in burnout among athletes so that future researchers may formulate hypotheses based on previous athlete burnout literature rather than the available coach research.

The results of the abovementioned research have left the burnout arena with several significant issues that warrant future attention. First, the relationship of decision-making style and burnout among coaches has yet to be clearly identified as research has yielded inconsistent findings. An additional issue of concern regards the incongruity between athlete and coach burnout and coaches' decision-making behaviors. Research has suggested that the decision-making style that has been linked to coach burnout (democratic or consideration) is one that may keep athletes from experiencing burnout. Further, the decision-making style linked to athlete burnout (autocratic) may be one that safeguards coaches from experiencing burnout. Additional research is needed to examine this relationship and ultimately reduce the potential of either group experiencing burnout. Further, the inconsistent results regarding gender differences in burnout among coaches and the paucity of research examining gender differences in burnout among athletes highlights the need for empirical research attention in both of these areas as well.

Therefore, the present research examined the relationship between perceived coaches' decision-making style and athletes' and coaches' burnout levels in the competitive sport of collegiate swimming. Secondary purposes included assessing gender differences in burnout within the coach and athlete populations, as well as the interaction between decision-making style and gender on burnout dimensions.

Both athlete and coach burnout was assessed utilizing the multidimensional theoretical framework established by Raedeke and Smith (2001), which defines burnout as a psychological syndrome of emotional/physical exhaustion, reduced sense of accomplishment, and sport devaluation (Raedeke, 1997; Raedeke & Smith, 2001). The multidimensional model of leadership (Chelladurai & Saleh, 1980) served as the theoretical framework for assessing coach and athlete perceptions of leadership behaviors, in particular, democratic and autocratic decision-making. A democratic decision-making style was defined as a style in which coaches permit participation by athletes in decisions regarding team goals, practice methods, and game tactics and strategies. An autocratic decision-making style was defined as a style in which a coach exercises independence in decision making and stresses their authority in dealing with their athletes (Chelladurai & Doherty, 1998; Chelladurai & Saleh, 1980).

It was hypothesized that as athletes perceive their coach's decision-making style to be more autocratic in nature, their own reported levels of burnout will increase. Further, as athletes perceive their coach's decision-making style to be democratic their own reported levels of burnout will decrease. Second, it was hypothesized that as coaches report more of autocratic style for decision-making their reported levels of burnout will decrease. Further, as coaches report more of a democratic decision-making style their reported levels of burnout will increase.

It was also hypothesized that male athletes who perceive more autocratic behaviors will report less burnout than their female counterparts. The same relationship was expected in the coaching population. It was also hypothesized that coaches who are high in autocratic behaviors and low in democratic behaviors will report less burnout than those coaches who are higher in democratic behaviors and lower in autocratic behaviors. Athletes who perceive their coaches to be higher in autocratic behaviors and lower in democratic behaviors will report more burnout than those athletes who report a perception of higher democratic and lower autocratic behaviors.

Methods

Participants

Athlete participants included male (n=38) and female (n=53) collegiate swimmers (N=91). Seventy-six collegiate swimmers competed in NCAA Division I (n=49) and Division II (n=27) programs. An additional 15 collegiate swimmers competing outside of NCAA governance also participated in the study. Athletes' ages ranged from 19 to 25 years with a mean age of 19.98 years (SD= 2.38). The average number of years athletes reported swimming competitively was 11.43 (SD=3.23). Athletes also reported spending an average of 20.93 hours per week on swimming-related obligations (SD=4.74).

The coaching sample included thirty-six collegiate swimming coaches who were affiliated with NCAA Division I (n=13), Division II (n=8), and Division III (n=9) swimming programs. Five coaches did not report their divisional status and one international collegiate swimming coach was employed outside of the United States. Twenty-three of the coaches were male and eight were female. Gender was not reported by five participants. The mean age of coach participants was 39.64 years (SD=9.94) with ages ranging from 23 to 58 years. The average number of years coaches reported coaching competitive swimming was 18.75 (SD=9.77). Coaches also reported spending an average of 50.28 hours per week on coaching-related duties (SD=16.82).

Measures Completed by Athletes

Swimmer Demographic Information Form. All collegiate swimmers completed a demographic information form that assessed personal characteristics, number of years swimming competitively, number of hours spent per week on swimming-related duties, and variables pertaining to their academic level and level of competition.

Athlete Burnout Questionnaire (ABQ). The Athlete Burnout Questionnaire (Raedeke & Smith, 2001) was used to assess levels of burnout in swimmers. This multidimensional inventory contains 15 items that assess three subscales of sport burnout: a) reduced sense of accomplishment, b) emotional and physical exhaustion, and c) sport devaluation. Participants respond to the degree each item applies to him or her using a Likert-type scale ranging from 1 ("almost never) to 5 ("almost always"). The psychometric properties of this instrument have been deemed adequate as construct validity and test-retest reliability were established during the inventory's construction (Raedeke & Smith, 2001).

Leadership Scale for Sports (LSS: Athlete Perception). To assess athletes' perceived decision-making style of their coaches, Chelladurai and Saleh's (1978, 1980) Leadership Scale for Sports was utilized. The LSS is a 40-item inventory that assesses several dimensions of coaches' leadership behaviors: a) social support, b) training and instruction, c) positive feedback, d) autocratic behavior, and e) democratic behavior. In completing the leadership perception inventory athletes are asked to respond by indicating how often their coach exhibits particular leadership behaviors. Their answers for each question are anchored from 1 ("always") to 5 ("never").

The psychometric properties of the LSS were demonstrated during its construction and included test-retest reliability (coefficients ranged from .71 to .82) and subscale internal consistencies (Chelladurai & Saleh, 1980). Cronbach's alpha coefficients for the five subscales were above .70 except the autocratic subscale. Because previous research has also found the autocratic subscale to have questionable internal consistency (Dwyer & Fischer, 1988) this component of the LSS was of concern for the present research. To compensate for the potential inadequate reliability of this subscale, improvements to its internal consistency were made based on previous research by Price and Weiss (2000). These authors added three items to the autocratic subscale for their study which resulted in adequate reliability for this subscale. These items were also used for the present study with those authors' permission.

Measures Completed by Coaches

Swimming Coach Demographic Information Form. All collegiate swimming coaches completed a demographic information form that assessed personal characteristics, number of years coaching swimming competitively, number of hours spent per week on swimming-related duties, and variables pertaining to their academic level and level of competition.

Coach Burnout Questionnaire (CBQ). Because there is no known sport-specific coaching burnout measure available to date, a modified version of the Athlete Burnout Questionnaire was developed to assess burnout levels in coaches. The principal investigator modified each of the 15 items in the original questionnaire to reflect coaching rather than playing their respective sport. For example, "I'm accomplishing many worthwhile things in swimming" was changed to "I'm accomplishing many worthwhile things in coaching swimming." After being modified, the coach version of the inventory was submitted to an expert panel of four former competitive swimmers and coaches/teachers who reviewed the original and modified version of the questionnaire and examined fit, clarity, and meaning of the revised items. No items were found by the panel to be inappropriately modified. This modified version appeared to have content validity and served as the Coach Burnout Questionnaire.

Leadership Scale for Sports (LSS: Coach Perception). The coach perception version of the LSS was used to assess coaches' perceptions of their own decision-making behaviors. The inventory was created along with the other versions of the scale using the same procedure previously described for the collegiate swimmer sample. Previous research has demonstrated adequate psychometric properties of this version of the LSS (Turman, 2003). To combat the potentially inadequate reliability of the autocratic subscale, the same additional three items that were added to the athlete perception version were also used for the coach perception version.

Procedures

Athletes. Data from collegiate swimmers were collected at the World Swimming Championships held in the Midwest United States. Those collegiate swimmers participating in or volunteering at the Championships who were willing to participate were given a counterbalanced packet containing a cover letter and the study's inventories and asked to place the forms in the envelope provided once completed. To increase the sample size of collegiate swimmers, additional data were collected from collegiate swimmers across collegiate athletic programs in the southeast region of the United States. Those collegiate swimmers who were willing to participate were given a counterbalanced packet containing the questionnaires and asked to place the inventories in an envelope once finished. Between both rounds of data collection, 22 athletes who were competing in the Championships were sampled. Sixty-nine collegiate swimmers not participating in the event were also sampled.

Coaches. Data from collegiate swimming coaches were collected at a world swimming coach's clinic held in the Midwest. Those collegiate swimming coaches willing to participate (n=25) were given a counterbalanced packet containing a cover letter and the study's inventories and asked to place the inventories in an envelope once finished. To increase the sample size of swimming coaches, additional data were obtained by uploading the coach inventories on the Internet under the domain of the university the researcher was affiliated with. With permission from the organization's director, members of a collegiate swimming coaches' organization received an e-mail explaining the purpose and procedures of the study in addition to a request for their participation. Those who were willing to complete the inventories (n=11) followed a link to a webpage containing electronic versions of the study's instruments for completion. Previous research has evaluated the psychometric equivalency of Internet-based research and found that data collection on the web is a valid and reliable method of acquiring data similar to that obtained when using traditional paper and pencil methods (Metzger, Kristof, & Yoest, 2003; Meyerson & Tryon, 2003).

Results

Preliminary Analyses for Collegiate Swimmers

To assess the reliability of the ABQ and LSS: Athlete Perception subscales, internal consistencies were calculated using Cronbach's alpha coefficients (See Table 1). All alpha coefficients were found to be above .70. Descriptive data for swimmers' perceptions of coaches' decision-making style for those subscales of the LSS in addition to their reported levels of burnout of each subscale of the ABQ can also be found in Table 1. The means for athletes' perception of their coach's decision-making style are comparable to those reported by Chelladurai (personal communication, March 1, 2004). An analysis of those studies using the athlete perception version of the LSS yielded an average democratic score of 3.05 (*SD*= .71) and an average mean for the autocratic scores of 2.64 (*SD*=.72). Norms for the ABQ are not yet available for comparison with the present study's results.

To examine any potential differences in the data obtained from those collegiate swimmers competing in the World Swimming Championships and those swimmers who did not compete in the event, independent sample *t*-tests were utilized. The only significant difference between the two groups of collegiate swimmers was on the democratic subscale of the LSS (t (89) = -2.5, $p<.05$).

Those competing in the Championships reported perceiving significantly more democratic behaviors of their coaches than did those swimmers not competing in the event. It should be noted, however, that the mean difference between group scores was .38 and was not deemed practically significant for the purposes of the present study. Therefore, both athletic groups were combined into one group for the purpose of subsequent data analyses.

Table 1. Internal consistency and descriptive statistics for intercollegiate swimmers (*N*=91) and coaches (*N*=36)

	Cronbach α	*M*	*SD*
ATHLETES			
ABQ			
Exhaustion	.91	3.06	.890
Sport Devaluation	.80	2.15	.803
Reduced Sense of Accomplishment	.79	2.15	.702
LSS			
Perceived Autocratic Behaviors	.80	2.76	.744
Perceived Democratic Behaviors	.81	3.30	.711
COACHES			
CBQ			
Exhaustion	.94	2.73	.984
Sport Devaluation	.88	2.03	.836
Reduced Sense of Accomplishment	.81	2.07	.671
LSS			
Perceived Autocratic Behaviors	.61	2.62	.470
Perceived Democratic Behaviors	.76	3.12	.492

Relationship between Perceived Decision-Making Style and Burnout among Swimmers

To examine the relationship between collegiate swimmers' perceived decision-making style of their coaches and their own reported levels of burnout, Pearson product-moment correlations were computed (see Table 2). The results revealed a statistically significant inverse relationship between swimmers' perception of a democratic decision-making style and their reported levels of burnout on all three subscales. Correlation coefficients ranged from r= -.28 to -.33 ($p<.01$). Results also revealed significant relationships between swimmers' perception of an autocratic decision-making style of their coaches and their reported levels of burnout on all three subscales. Correlation coefficients from this analysis ranged from r= .22 to .32 ($p<.05$).

Table 2. Pearson product correlation coefficients for burnout and decision-making style among collegiate swimmers (*N*=91) and collegiate swimming coaches (*N*=36)

	Autocratic	Democratic
ATHLETES		
Exhaustion	.25*	-.28**
Sport Devaluation	.32**	-.33**
Reduced Sense of Accomplishment	.22*	-.28**
COACHES		
Exhaustion	.02	-.11
Sport Devaluation	-.11	-.02
Reduced Sense of Accomplishment	-.24	.11

*p<.05
**p<.01

Gender, Autocratic Decision-Making Style, and Burnout among Swimmers

To assess interactions between collegiate swimmers' gender and a perceived coaches' autocratic decision-making style on their burnout levels, three, two-way (gender x high/low autocratic) ANOVAs were utilized. Each burnout subscale served as a dependent variable for the ANOVAs conducted. Collegiate swimmers' scores on the perceived autocratic decision-making behavior subscale of the LSS were recoded into either high or low autocratic perception categories. A median split was used to determine if scores were categorized as high or low. Those scores above the median were classified as high autocratic perception and those below classified as low autocratic perception.

The results of the ANOVAs revealed no statistically significant interactions between gender and autocratic perceptions of collegiate swimmers on any of the three subscales of burnout. Further examination revealed no significant main effects for gender or high/low autocratic perception on any of the three burnout subscales.

Gender, Democratic Decision-Making Style, and Burnout among Swimmers

Three, two-way (gender x high/low democratic) ANOVAs were also computed to examine any interactions between collegiate swimmers' gender and a perceived coaches' democratic decision-making style on these athletes' own levels of burnout. Again, each burnout subscale was used as a dependent variable. Swimmers' scores on the perceived democratic decision-making behavior subscale of the LSS were recoded as being either a high or low democratic perception. Similar to the autocratic scale, a median split was used to determine if scores were categorized as high or low.

The results of the ANOVAs revealed no significant interactions between gender and democratic perceptions of collegiate swimmers on any of the three burnout subscales. No significant main effects were found for gender on any of the burnout subscales. However, a significant main effect was found for perceptions of democratic behaviors with regard to the exhaustion burnout subscale (F (1, 87) = 6.13, p<.05, η^2=.07). Those swimmers perceiving their coach to use a high degree of democratic decision-making behaviors reported significantly less emotional and physical exhaustion than those reporting their coaches to be less democratic. A significant main effect was also found for perceptions of democratic behaviors regarding the sport devaluation burnout subscale (F (1, 87) = 7.23, p<.01, η^2= .08). Collegiate swimmers perceiving their coach as using a high degree of democratic decision-making behaviors reported significantly less sport devaluation than those swimmers reporting their coaches to be less democratic.

The Influence of Both Decision-Making Styles on Swimmers' Burnout

Three, two-way (high/low autocratic x high/low democratic) ANOVAs were also computed to examine any interactions between both decision-making styles and burnout among collegiate swimmers. Again, each burnout subscale was used as a dependent variable. Swimmers' scores on the perceived democratic and autocratic decision-making behavior subscales of the LSS were recoded as being either a high or low perception. A median split was again used to determine if scores were categorized as high or low.

The results revealed no significant interactions between both decision-making styles on collegiate swimmers' levels of burnout. Significant main effects were found for the democratic subscales on the exhaustion (F (1, 87) = 5.73, p<.05, η^2= .06) and sport devaluation (F (1, 87)= 5.52, p<.05, η^2= .06) burnout subscales. Collegiate swimmers perceiving their coaches to use a higher degree of democratic decision-making behaviors reported significantly less burnout on these subscales than those swimmers reporting a low perception of democratic decision-making behaviors.

Does Perception of Decision-Making Style Predict Burnout among Swimmers?

Because it was hypothesized that collegiate swimmers' perception of their coach's decision-making style would influence their own reported levels of burnout, it was logical to ascertain the predictive value of decision-making style on swimmers' burnout. To examine this, three stepwise multiple regression analyses were conducted. Each burnout subscale served as one of the criterion variables. To determine if any additional demographic predictor variables should be included in the analyses, in addition to testing for multicolinearity, a Pearson product-moment correlation matrix was utilized. The results revealed no significant relationships between athletes' demographic information (e.g. number of years swimming competitively, number of hours per week spent on swimming-related duties) and any of the three burnout subscales. Therefore, no additional demographic variables were included in the regression analyses. Neither predictor variables (autocratic decision-making style, democratic decision-making style) were found to be highly correlated with one another suggesting multicolinearity was not of concern.

The only statistically significant predictor of the emotional and physical exhaustion component of burnout was the perception of a democratic decision-making style (F (1, 89) =7.39, p<.01). This model was only found to account for just under 8% of the variance in the exhaustion burnout subscale (R^2=.078). Two models were found to account for a statistically significant amount of the variance in the sport devaluation subscale of burnout. The most parsimonious of the two found perceptions of both a democratic and autocratic decision-making style to be significant predictors of depersonalization (F (2, 89) =8.49, p<.001). This model, while significant, only accounted for about 16% of the variance in the criterion variable (R^2=.163). For the reduced sense of accomplishment subscale of burnout, a model containing only a perception of democratic decision-making behaviors accounted for a statistically significant amount of the variance (F (1,89) =7.25, p<.01). This model was found to account for only about 7% of the variance (R^2= .076).

Preliminary Analyses for Collegiate Swimming Coaches

To assess the reliability of the CBQ and LSS: Coach Perception subscales, internal consistencies were calculated using Cronbach's alpha coefficients (See Table 1). Reliability coefficients ranged from .80 to .93 for the three burnout subscales. Cronbach's alpha coefficients for the perceptions of democratic and autocratic decision-making behaviors were lower. This was particularly true for the autocratic subscale for which its low reliability has been reported in previous research (Dwyer & Fischer, 1988).

Descriptive data for swimming coaches' perceptions of each decision-making style in addition to their reported levels of burnout can also be found in Table 1. Coaches in the present study reported using significantly more democratic than autocratic behaviors. These results are similar to those found by Dwyer and Fischer (1988) whose sample of wrestling coaches yielded a comparable pattern.

To examine any differences between coaches surveyed via paper and pencil questionnaires at the swimming coaching clinic and those coaches completing inventories over the Internet, independent samples *t*-tests were utilized. The results revealed no significant mean score differences between the two groups on any of the inventories' subscales. Therefore, both groups of data were combined for subsequent analyses.

Relationship between Perceived Decision-Making Style and Burnout among Coaches

To examine the relationship between collegiate swimmers coaches' perceived decision-making style and their own reported levels of burnout, Pearson product-moment correlations were computed (see Table 2). The results revealed no statistically significant relationships between the perception of possessing an autocratic or democratic decision-making style and coaches' scores on any of the three burnout subscales.

Gender, Decision-Making Style, and Burnout among Coaches

To assess any differences in collegiate swimming coaches' gender on their burnout levels, three independent *t*-tests were utilized. Each burnout subscale served as a dependent variable. No significant differences were found between males and females on any of the burnout subscales.

To examine differences in burnout between coaches categorized as using high versus low levels of democratic or autocratic decision-making behaviors, six additional independent *t*-tests were utilized. Three *t*-test analyses were computed for each decision-making style, one for each of the three burnout subscales serving as the dependent variable. Collegiate swimming coaches' scores on their perceived autocratic and democratic decision-making behavior subscales of the LSS were recoded into either high or low perceptions. A median split was used to determine if scores were categorized as high or low. No significant differences were found on any of the three burnout subscales between those coaches classified as using a high or low degree of democratic or autocratic decision-making behaviors.

Discussion

The Influence of Decision-Making Style on Collegiate Swimmers' Burnout

The primary purpose of the present research was to examine the relationship between the perceived decision-making style of coaches and burnout among coaches and athletes. The most significant finding was the link established between collegiate swimmers' perception of their coach's decision-making style and their own reported levels of burnout. As hypothesized for the athlete sample, collegiate swimmers' levels of burnout on all three subscales were significantly related to their perception of coaches' use of autocratic and democratic decision-making styles. As swimmers perceived their coach to utilize more of an autocratic decision-making style, swimmers' reported levels of burnout on all three subscales increased. Further, as swimmers perceived their coach to utilize more of a democratic decision-making style, their reported levels of burnout on all three subscales decreased.

The relationships between swimmers' perceived decision-making style of their coach and their reported level of burnout were further confirmed by the results of the two-way ANOVAs and regression analyses. Collegiate swimmers perceiving their coaches to be more democratic in their decision-making reported significantly less burnout on these subscales than those swimmers' perceiving their coaches to use fewer democratic decision-making behaviors. In addition, perception of decision-making style was found to significantly predict all three subscales of burnout among collegiate swimmers. Collectively, these results suggest that collegiate swimmers' perception of their coach's decision-making style, particularly a democratic style of decision-making, has some influence on swimmers' reported levels of burnout.

The results of the swimmers' data mirror those of previous research examining the influences of coach leadership on athlete burnout within a multidimensional model of leadership (e.g. Price & Weiss, 2000; Vealey et al., 1998). Because democratic coaches elicit feedback from their athletes regarding decisions about their team, these athletes may perceive to have more control over and meaning in their sport participation. These perceptions may help act as a buffer against the physical and psychological stressors that, over time, can eventually lead to burnout. Contrastingly, autocratic coaches do not invite feedback from their athletes. This could contribute to a lack of perceived control and meaning among athletes regarding their sport involvement and could partially contribute to an extreme training environment that Vealey et al. (1998) noted athletes cite as the most significant cause of burnout. The results also support the findings of Udry and colleagues (1997), that suggested athletes coping with burnout often view their sport interactions with important others (including coaches) as more negative than positive. The perception of an autocratic decision-making style of their coach could contribute to collegiate swimmers' negative perception of "important others."

It is of interest that swimmers' perception of a democratic decision-making style emerged from the analyses as the more salient of the two types of decision-making styles linked to burnout levels in swimmers. A likely explanation for this finding may rest in the type of sport used for the present research. Weinberg and Gould (2007) noted that athletes participating in interactive, team sports may prefer more of an autocratic style of decision-making than athletes taking part in a coactive sport such as swimming. Partially due to the nature of their sport, swimmers' responses to the inventories may have reflected the preference for a democratic style which would help explain why more democratic than autocratic behaviors were reported by both swimmers and swimming coaches.

The secondary purposes of the present research were to examine the influence of gender and decision-making style on collegiate swimmers' burnout, in addition to the interaction of both decision-making styles on swimmers' burnout. It was hypothesized that male collegiate swimmers perceiving their coach to utilize more autocratic decisions would report less burnout than females. The results of the analyses did not support this hypothesis. Further, collegiate swimmers did not significantly differ between genders on their level of burnout on any of the three subscales. Although males have been found to prefer an autocratic style of decision-making more than females (Chelladurai & Saleh, 1978; Chelladurai & Carron, 1983; Turman, 2003), it may be that this preference does little to influence the prevalence of burnout among male versus female athletes. The failure to reveal significant gender differences in burnout among athletes does, however, support previous research conducted by Lai and Wiggins (2003). In conducting their research, these authors utilized coach burnout research to formulate their hypotheses regarding gender differences. Because little research has examined gender differences in burnout among athletes, it is important that future studies do so in the hopes that such hypotheses can be made using the results of athlete data rather than that of coaches.

It was also of interest that the two decision-making styles did not interact significantly to influence burnout among collegiate swimmers. This suggests that for the collegiate swimmers and swimming coaches surveyed, a particular combination of both decision-making styles did not influence the degree of burnout either group experienced. Prior to this study, research had not examined the potential interaction between these two distinct leadership characteristics.

The Influence of Decision-Making Style on Collegiate Swimming Coaches' Burnout

Another purpose of this study was also to examine the relationship between coaches' perception of their decision-making style and coaches' reported levels of burnout. It was hypothesized that as collegiate swimming coaches perceived themselves to utilize more of a democratic style of decision-making, their reported levels of burnout would increase. Further, as these coaches reported more of an autocratic style of decision-making, their levels of burnout would decrease. The results of the analyses did not support this hypothesis; collegiate swimming coaches' perception of their decision-making style was not found to be significantly related to any of the three burnout subscales. Subsequent analyses confirmed this finding as coaches classified as being high in their use of autocratic or democratic decision-making behaviors did not significantly differ from one another on any of the three burnout subscales. There were no differences in burnout revealed between male and female coaches as well. Finally, perception of decision-making style did not significantly predict burnout in collegiate swimming coaches.

Several propositions can be offered in understanding why these results emerged. One must acknowledge the possibility that coaches responded to the questionnaires in a socially desirable manner. In fact, previous research has masked the true nature of burnout questionnaires to account for the negative connotation associated with the construct of burnout (e.g. Gould, Udry, Tuffey, & Loehr, 1996b). The lack of willingness among coaches to express their true levels of burnout and style of decision-making could have potentially contributed to the findings of the present study.

The accuracy of the coaches' responses to the study's questionnaires, particularly the LSS, may also be worthy of consideration. Research has found that coaches' perceptions of their own leadership behaviors are less accurate than those of the athletes they coach (Smoll & Smith, 1981). It is possible that a portion of coaches sampled in the present study misrepresented their decision-making behaviors on the LSS due to an inaccurate perception of those behaviors, which could influence the results of the analyses conducted on the swimming coaches' data.

The failure to reveal gender differences among coaches on any of the three burnout subscales is not surprising when one takes into consideration the equivocal findings of previous research (Davenport, 1998). Caccese and Mayerberg (1984) found that female coaches experienced significantly higher levels of burnout denoted by greater levels of emotional exhaustion and lower levels of personal accomplishments than their male counterpart. Similar results have been found in other studies regarding the emotional exhaustion subscale (Kelley, 1994; Kelley et al., 1999; Pastore & Judd, 1993; Vealey et al., 1992) with others unable to demonstrate gender differences among the personal accomplishment subscale (Pastore & Judd, 1993; Vealey et al., 1992). Where some have found no gender differences in depersonalization, other researchers have suggested males experience greater levels of depersonalization than females (Dale & Weinberg, 1989). Additional research is clearly warranted that targets the potential gender differences among both coaches and athletes.

Finally, one has to consider the reported levels of burnout by both athletes and coaches in the present study. The sample of collegiate swimmers and swimming coaches obtained were not experiencing a high degree of burnout. Further, because the ABQ and CBQ are newer instruments used in the assessment of sport burnout, norms are not available for comparison. It is possible that many of the swimmers participating in the study, particularly those swimmers competing in the Championships, were surveyed immediately following a tapering period of their training in preparation for this significant competition. Because these athletes had not recently been exposed to the extreme training conditions that swimmers typically endure, their reported levels of burnout may have been slightly lower.

Implications and Future Directions

The results of the present research revealed that collegiate swimmers' perception of their coaches' decision-making style has some degree of influence on burnout levels reported by those swimmers. Thus, it could be suggested that coaches take into consideration the degree to which they elicit feedback from their athletes regarding team-related decisions. By eliciting feedback from athletes, coaches could help create a feeling of control and meaningfulness among athletes that act as a buffer against experiencing burnout. This idea is further supported by the fact that results did not show collegiate swimming coaches' decision-making style was related to or predictive of coach burnout. Coaches who utilize a democratic style of decision-making with their team might help prevent burnout among their players without enhancing their own likelihood of experiencing the same.

Future burnout research should continue to examine the relationship between coaches' leadership variables and their impact on both coach and athlete burnout. A useful approach would be to incorporate qualitative research methods in burnout investigations of coaches and athletes experiencing a high degree of burnout as has been done in the past (e.g. Gould, Tuffey, Udry, & Loehr, 1996a). This would be particularly helpful with a coach population, as little qualitative burnout research has been done with this group.

Additional research attention should also be given to the assessment of burnout within the sport domain. Because the ABQ was developed recently, norms for the subscales and additional validation of the instrument have yet to be provided. The present research provided additional support for the internal consistency of this measure, although future research should continue to validate its psychometric properties across various sport types and establish norms for each of its subscales to compare future research with. The present research also provided preliminary support for a measure to assess sport burnout in coaches. To date, no sport burnout measure is available for the coach population. The internal consistencies found with the CBQ were high and a promising indication that such a measure could be developed and validated.

References

Caccese, T., & Mayerberg, C. (1984). Gender differences in perceived burnout of college coaches. *Journal of Sport Psychology, 6,* 279-288.

Chelladurai, P. (1984). Discrepancy between preferences and perceptions of leadership behavior and satisfaction of athletes in varying sports. *Journal of Sport Psychology, 6,* 27-41.

Chelladurai, P., & Carron, A.V. (1983). Athletic maturity and preferred leadership. *Journal of Sport Psychology, 5,* 371-380.

Chelladurai, P., & Doherty, A. (1998). Styles of decision making in coaching. In J. Williams (Ed.), *Applied sport psychology: Personal growth to peak performance* (pp.115-126). Mountain View, CA: Mayfield Publishing Company.

Chelladurai, P., & Saleh, S.D. (1978). Preferred leadership in sports. *Canadian Journal of Applied Sport Sciences, 3,* 85-92.

Chelladurai, P., & Saleh, S.D. (1980). Dimensions of leader behavior in sports: Development of a leadership scale. *Journal of Sport Psychology, 2,* 34-45.

Dale, J., & Weinberg, R. (1989). The relationship between coaches' leadership style and burnout. *The Sport Psychologist, 3,* 1-13.

Davenport, M. (1998). *A descriptive analysis of the burnout of rowing coaches over a competitive season.* Unpublished doctoral dissertation, Wilmington College, Wilmington, Ohio.

Dwyer, J., & Fischer, D. (1988). Psychometric properties of the coach's version of Leadership Scale for Sports. *Perceptual and Motor Skills, 67,* 795-798.

Gould, D., Tuffey, S., Udry, E., & Loehr, J. (1996a). Burnout in competitive junior tennis players: II. A qualitative analysis. *The Sport Psychologist, 10,* 341-366.

Gould, D., Udry, E., Tuffey, S., & Loehr, J. (1996b). Burnout in competitive junior tennis players: I. A quantitative psychological assessment. *The Sport Psychologist, 10,* 322-340.

Kelley, B. (1994). A model of stress and burnout in collegiate coaches: Effects of gender and time of seascn. *Research Quarterly for Exercise and Sport, 65,* 48-58.

Kelley, B., Eklund, R., & Ritter-Taylor, M. (1999). Stress and burnout among collegiate tennis coaches. *Journal of Sport and Exercise Psychology, 21,* 113-130.

Lai, C., & Wiggins, S. (2003). Burnout perceptions over time in NCAA division I soccer players. *International Sports Journal, 7,* 120-127.

Maslach, C., & Jackson, S. (1981). The measurement of experienced burnout. *Journal of Occupational Behaviour, 2,* 99-113.

Metzger, M., Kristof, V., & Yoest, D. (2003). The world wide web and the laboratory: A comparison using face recognition. *Cyberpsychology and Behavior: The Impact of the Internet, Multimedia, and Virtual Reality on Behavior and Society, 6,* 613-621.

Meyerson, P., & Tryon, W. (2003). Validating internet research: A test of the psychometric equivalence of Internet and in-person samples. *Behavior Research Methods, Instruments and Computers, 35,* 614-620.

Pastore, D., & Judd, M. (1993). Gender differences in burnout among coaches of women's athletic teams at 2-year colleges. *Sociology of Sport Journal, 10,* 205-212.

Price, M., & Weiss, M. (2000). Relationships among coach burnout, coach behaviors, and athletes' psychological responses. *The Sport Psychologist, 14,* 391-409.

Raedeke, T. (1997). Is athlete burnout more than just stress? A sport commitment perspective. *Journal of Sport and Exercise Psychology, 19,* 396-417.

Raedeke, T., & Smith, A. (2001). Development and preliminary validation of an athlete burnout measure. *Journal of Sport and Exercise Psychology, 23,* 281-306.

Smoll, F., & Smith, R. (1981). Preparation of youth sport coaches: An educational application of sport psychology. *Physical Educator, 38,* 85-94.

Turman, P. (2003). Athletic coaching from an instructional communication perspective: The influence of coach experience on high school wrestlers' preferences and perceptions of coaching behaviors across a season. *Communication Education, 52,* 73-86.

Udry, E., Gould, D., Bridges, D., & Tuffey, S. (1997). People helping people? Examining the social ties of athletes coping with burnout and injury stress. *Journal of Sport and Exercise Psychology, 19,* 368-395.

Vealey, R., Armstrong, L., Comar, W., & Greenleaf, C. (1998). Influence of perceived coaching behaviors on burnout and competitive anxiety in female college athletes. *Journal of Applied Sport Psychology, 10,* 297-318.

Vealey, R., Udry, E., Zimmerman, V., & Soliday, J. (1992). Intrapersonal and situational predictors of coaching burnout. *Journal of Sport and Exercise Psychology, 14,* 40-58.

Weinberg, R., & Gould, D. (2007). *Foundations of sport and exercise psychology.* Champaign, IL: Human Kinetics.

Index

A

B

C

D

E

F

G

H

I

J

K

L

Q

R

S

W

Y